TABLE OF CONTENTS

INTRODUCTION

CHAPTER 1: MEANING AND BASICS OF REFLEXOLOGY

CHAPTER 2: REFLEXOLOGY BASICS

CHAPTER 3: REFLEXOLOGY BENEFITS

CHAPTER 4: SOME TIPS TO BEAR IN MIND WHILE PRACTICING REFLEXOLOGY

CHAPTER 5: TYPES OF REFLEXOLOGY

CHAPTER 6: REFLEXOLOGY AND BODY BALANCE

CHAPTER 7: SPORTS REFLEXOLOGY

CHAPTER 8: GETTING A DEGREE AND STARTING YOUR BUSINESS

CHAPTER 9: PRECAUTIONS TO BEAR IN MIND

CHAPTER 10: WHO CAN IT HELP?

CHAPTER 11: TRAINING AND EDUCATION

CONCLUSION

FREE BONUS

INTRODUCTION

In this day and age where everybody leads a hectic life, it becomes all the more important to find a way to relax and recoil. One effective method that can be used to achieve the same is "reflexology".

Therapists from the West have discovered methods to not only influence and create balance from energies that radiate through the body and escapes from the hands and feet, but mastered the techniques. The therapy, in relation to energy, has become widely popular among a reflexology session. What is this new trend of treatment? It is associated with the massaging of the body in order to relieve tension through the reflex points. These points are located through either the head, feet or hands.

Gentle grasps of the reflexes can be linked together to create a balance of energy within the body. Oils and magnets are applications that are able to be applied to these sensitive areas, hands, feet, forehead and scalp. Ears are becoming a widely popular addition to the use of foot reflexology. In most cases, the client can have all three areas worked on in one session. It is clearly opinion and how the client responds to the therapy.

Reflexology isn't practiced in such the regions just of the west, it is all over the world, such as Australia

Those therapists are training with different methods and techniques to fit the needs of specific clients, the disabled, the impaired, and sometimes mentally ill.

ORIGINS OF REFLEXOLOGY

It is well known that the healing art known as reflexology has its roots back in ancient times. Although we do not know where and when the art began, the earliest evidence we have is from wall reliefs located within an ancient Egyptian tomb from the Sixth Dynasty (c. 2450 BCE) which show two men having their hands and feet massaged. It then appears that this type of practice was transferred into the classical world, both in ancient Greece and Rome. We also see evidence of an early form of reflexology in ancient China, to around 3000 BCE and also in ancient India. There may be evidence of it practiced in the Incan culture and possibly found its way to the Native Americans who lived in contemporary USA.

Due to its ancient roots, tracing the history and its actual origins is somewhat difficult for us. It is believed, however, that the art of reflexology was passed down from one generation to the next by verbal means long before it was painted on the Egyptian walls of the tomb of Ankhamor in the Sixth Dynasty in addition to other illustrations of various medical practices. In ancient Egypt, archaeologists discovered illustrations of certain points on the foot and being linked to certain internal organs. The ancient Egyptian doctors believed that the human body was made up of a symphony of vibrations. Through applying pressure on particular locations upon the foot, they believed that the organs could be played right.

In India and then China, there have been a number of symbols relating to reflexology located on the feet of statues of Buddha from various points in history. There is a chapter in the ancient Chinese medical text, The Yellow Emperor's Classic of Internal Medicine, which tells of "Examining Foot Method" which tells of certain areas of the foot relating to the life force of the person. This is dated to around 1000 BCE.

In the 14th century, it is believed that the Venetian explorer, Marco Polo, had a book on Chinese massage translated into Italian and then brought the conception and practice of reflexology and massage into western Europe. Then in 1582, Dr. Adamus and Dr. A'tatis published a book on the essential component of reflexology which they termed zone therapy.

In the early 20th century, Dr. Willian H. Fitzgerald of the United States published a work regarding 10 vertical zones that ran up and down the entire body. He discovered that when you applied pressure to one of these zones then it related to a location of where an injury was and that it could help relieve pain whilst undergoing minor surgeries. This was published in 1917 and Fitzgerald is referred to as the father of modern reflexology.

His research on reflexology was then enhanced by a Dr. Shelby Riley who then created a map of a series of horizontal lines and a meticulous map of points corresponding to areas on both the hands and feet. Riley also proposed certain points located on the outer part of the ear.

When we look at the practice of reflexology in modern times, we can see that it has had a deep impact on many western cultures. In the latter part of the 19th century in the United Kingdom, Sir Henry Head was the first to research into the notions behind reflexology. Around this time, scholars in Germany and Russia were looking into the practice themselves, although there were different reasons behind their own studies.

Within 20 years, it was Fitzgerald (previously mentioned) that put forward his theories of zones which he termed zone analgesia or zone therapy. His lines began from the hands and the feet. His theories were published as Relieving Pain at Home.

It would be a physical therapist named Eunice D. Ingham who would really put the healing art soon to be known as reflexology on the map. In the 1930s, Ingham studied the concept of the healing art and found that the pressure points on the feet were located in a reverse image of the relating organs of the body where the corresponding points were identified. Her discovery was published within the Stories the Feet Can Tell, which was published in 1938. Her work was initially referred by some people as zone therapy on closer inspection there are differences within the two therapies of pressure analgesia. One particular difference is that reflexology describes a specific association between the pressure points and the afflicted locations of the body. In addition to this, Ingham separated the foot into 12 specific areas whereas Fitzgerald divided the entire body into 10 vertical areas in his own theory.

In 1968, Dwight Byers and Eusebia Messenger, siblings, went on to found the National Institute of Reflexology but by the next decade it had expanded and was renamed as the International Institute of Reflexology.

EUNICE INGHAM 1889 – 1974

Born on the 24th February, Eunice Ingham grew up to become a physical therapist by trade. She worked alongside Dr. Shelby Riley who went on to publish his version of an active zone therapy, which was a separate therapy from reflexology although it did share certain characteristics. When she discovered a distinctive pattern of pressure and reflex points based on the feet, she concentrated on this to publish her own theories of reflexology before she eventually died in 1974, on the 10th of December.

Throughout her lifetime, Ingham would travel across the country and talk to audiences regarding reflexology. To begin with, the majority of her audience was the elderly or the infirm that were desperate to find any kind of relief from physical pain. But, as a result of finding an improvement in their conditions, her theory of reflexology began to catch the attention of other people, especially in the medical and scientific world, and became a respected therapy. In her published works, Stories the Feet Can Tell, she produces a map of the pressure points located on the human foot and their corresponding internal organs. This book went on to be published into 7 languages, although it was referred to as Zone Therapy in various places. It was this error which led to the original character of reflexology being mixed up with zone therapy instead of a therapy all by itself.

During her career, Ingham went on to practice her therapy on many patients with her identifying every part of the pressure points meticulously and would double check these areas until she was confident that she knew where each reflex point was and that there was an image on the organs located within the body.

It was her ultimate goal to help people through her notion of reflexology. She died when she was 85 years old after a lifetime of helping others. Her nephew, Dwight, went on to continue her work and would perform lectures about the benefits of reflexology. His daughter and then his grandson, continue her work even today.

Reflexology is both an art and a science and one of the most practiced forms of alternate therapies in the world.

It is a great little tool that you can use to avail relief from various body conditions such as fatigue, joint pains and other internal issues. The principles of reflexology are simple to understand and simpler to implement.

With a little knowledge on the basics, you will be able to practice it and avail its full benefits.

However, you must know that Reflexology is not a medicine or a surgery; it is more of a massage practice that helps in providing relief from aches and side effects caused by medicines and illnesses.

It is also widely used in the world of sports, where athletes are massaged using reflexology to provide instant relief.

In this book, we will look at the basics of reflexology and also the different techniques that you can use to avail relief from muscle tension.

I thank you for choosing this book and hope you have a good time reading it.

Let's get started!

CHAPTER 1

MEANING AND BASICS OF REFLEXOLOGY

In this first chapter, we will look at the basics of reflexology and understand its core concepts.

MEANING

Reflexology stands for the art of massaging and stimulating certain pressure points on the body that are individually connected to the different organs. As you know, the human body is all inter connected and it is possible for us to stimulate an internal organ by pressing over a point externally.

If you have heard of acupressure, then you will know how it works. The acupressurist stimulates the internal organs by pressing over certain pulse points that are placed externally. They will have extensive knowledge of what needs to be stimulated in order to massage the organ internally. The main concept of reflexology centers on "reflex" actions that the body parts experience when they are stimulated. Say for example you feel pain in your neck; the reflexologist will know a corresponding point under your foot, which upon stimulation will help in reliving the neck pain.

Similarly, they will know where to massage or apply pressure based on where the pain lies.

HISTORY

Reflexology is said to have its roots in a form a therapy known as zone therapy. As per zone therapy, the body is divided into 10 zones. These zones are all over the body. Each zone runs its length and ends in your fingertips or toes. So, by stimulating these points, you will be able to massage the internal organ effectively. However, you must first understand the basics of these zones before you can go about massaging or pressurizing these points. Here is how you can reach the internal organs based on where the individual points lie.

Zone 1 is connected to the toe and you will be able to control the entire zone by stimulating it. Similarly, zone 2 is connected with your second finger and you can stimulate the entire zone by pressurizing it and so on.

You can look up an online chart to see which point corresponds to which organ in the body. The chart will also tell you what the individual zones are and how you can stimulate them. You should understand that these points are highly sensitive and if you wish to stimulate them then you should exercise precaution.

After the zone system gained popularity, many ancient physicians and alternate therapists worked on the practice and bettered it. It is believed that its roots lie in ancient Egypt. Several hieroglyphs have been found on the tombs in Egypt that indicate the presence and spread of the practice of reflexology. It is then said to have travelled to china, where the Buddhists started practicing the art. Several statues and pictures of Buddha have been depicted as practicing reflexology.

In fact, reflexology was extensively covered in a book on alternate medicine that was released in 1000 BC. It was termed as the Examining foot technique and meant to help in relieving internal aches by stimulating pressure points based under the foot. The art then moved to India, where some additional features were introduced that complemented the existing art of reflexology. When Marco Polo visited Asia, he is said to have found the practice extremely useful and decided to write a book on it in the Italian language. This made it easy for Europeans to take up and exploit the practice.

Finally, in 1917, an American doctor, William H Fitzgerald took up the art form and exploited it. He is said to have coined the term and also delved deep into the details of reflexology.

Subsequently, Doctor Riley is said to have come up with a map of the different points that lie under the feet. He also made a map of the points that lie in the palm and the outside of the ear.

This map made it quite easy for people to know which points need to be stimulated in order to reach the different internal organs.

Other noteworthy names from the world of reflexology are that of Eunice Ingham and Doctor Nogier, both of whom are said to have conducted intense research on the topic and to whom modern day reflexology is attributed. Once reflexology was accepted as an alternate form of therapy, many therapists started subjecting their patients to it. Soon word of it started reaching the four corners of the globe and the practice garnered a therapeutic reputation.

People began using it to avail relief from stress and tensions. Soon, many massage centers began cropping up where people could avail the benefits of reflexology. More and more people began to avail the practice and also attracted the likes of sportsmen, athletes and celebrities. Reflexology today is more of a relaxant that people use to help relax their bodies.

Through the course of this book, we will look at the different techniques that are used in reflexology and how you can start with the practice at the earliest.

CHAPTER 2

REFLEXOLOGY BASICS

By now you must have understood what reflexology is all about and what it is mainly used for.

When it comes to understanding a subject, it is important to know what some of its basic concepts stand for. In this chapter, we will look at some of the basics of reflexology to help you understand the topic better.

WHAT TO EXPECT FROM A TYPICAL REFLEXOLOGY SESSION

Reflexology is a great way to relax and help relieve pain. It is a form of massage that depends greatly on the manipulation of pressure points using the therapist's hand. At times, reflexologists use oil to help ease the tension on their own hands, wrists and arms that builds up throughout a session. They try to choose oils that are beneficial to their patient, like sesame oil, aromatherapy oils and menthol.

The typical reflexology session can last about half of an hour, even though it can last up to an hour. The patient sits in a reclined position or on a medical table.

Luckily for people who are ticklish, the pressure that is applied during the session is firm, and is not feathery. So you do not have to worry as much about having a tickle response.

The amount of pressure that is used in each pressure point should be dictated by the patient. If the pressure is too light, the therapy will not work. If it is too heavy, the session will be painful.

Keep in mind; you do not have to be licensed to provide reflexology, as long as you only give medical advice that stays within the realm of reflexology. You cannot guarantee that reflexology is a cure or treatment for any specific type of illness or ailment. You can however tell patients that the form of relaxation provided by reflexology can aid in the treatment of these ailments.

You must also avoid giving your "medical opinion" about conditions. Always tell them that the best way to get information about their specific condition is to consult with their medical doctor.

Reflexology cannot be used by everyone. It cannot be used by those who have skin problems or circulatory irregularities. People who have had previous hand or foot trauma should not use reflexology either. This can cause serious accidents to happen during the session, which could result in displacement of nerve endings, or uncomfortable sensations.

AYURVEDIC REFLEXOLOGY: BLENDING WESTERN AND INDIAN REFLEXOLOGY METHODS

The art of reflexology goes back thousands of years. Even though it has an origin, there are so many methods that they have started to blend together. Historical accounts show that reflexology was used by Egyptians, Chinese, Japanese, and Indians. Since then, it has spread across the world and become one of the most beloved methods of treatment.

In India, the version of reflexology used is called Ayurvedic Reflexology. The people who practice this method do not call it such, they simply call it reflexology. It is a method that was born from using two separate principles of treatment, Ayurveda and reflexology.

Ayurveda is a blend of two separate Indian words, 'Ayur' meaning of life, and 'veda' meaning knowledge. Roughly translated, the term means 'the knowledge of life.' It is a treatment that involves the entire human body, including the mind, body and spirit. Unless there is a proper balance between the three, Indian beliefs do not feel as though balance and health can be obtained.

Ayurveda encourages the use of herbal medicine to help build a harmonious bond with nature. The herbs that are used focus on preventing illness and not actually curing anything specific.

Ayurvedic Reflexology insists that the best method of treatment is a daily massage followed by focusing on the pressure points that are associated with the imbalances that are felt by the person who is being treated.

Sesame oil is used as a lubricant to prevent friction during the reflexology session. It also helps to prevent injury to the reflexologists arm and wrist that are caused by repeated movement.

Whether you choose to utilize standard reflexology or Ayurvedic Reflexology, it must be used properly and the condition of the person's hands and feet must be taken into account before starting any session.

Most medical procedures are recommended to only be carried out by a qualified medical professional. They cannot be completed by the average person and some of them can be flat out dangerous if you try to practice them at home.

Reflexology, on the other hand, unlike many medical procedures is perfectly safe for almost anyone to understand and practice. It is a very effective, safe method of relieving pain and regaining a healthy, energetic balance.

Reflexology also knows no boundaries. It can be practiced on people from any age, of any sex, at any time. It is not dangerous, even if it is done completely wrong. Essentially, by trying reflexology for the first time, you have nothing to lose.

THE ZONE THEORY

The concept of zone therapy is the basis of reflexology. Every single body has a group of ten invisible life force currents that course through it. There are five life forces on the right side of the body, and five life forces on the left side. These life forces run from your head, to your feet.

The specific area that each life force falls under is considered a zone. All ten zones run down the body and cover every aspect, including the face, head, shoulders, arms, hands, chest, abdomen, reproductive organs, legs and feet.

Imagine, if you would, a human standing in front of you, palms facing forward, toes facing forward. There is a dividing line down the center of their body, extending from their head to their feet.

REFLEX POINTS IN THE HANDS

Part of the hand/foot   **Reflex Point**

Part of the hand/foot	Reflex Point
Big toes/thumbs	head/neck
Little toes/fingers	Head
Shoulder line to diaphragm line	Chest, lungs, shoulders
Arch (upper portion)	Diaphragm to waist portion of the body and the organs falling in the upper abdominal area
Arch (lower portion)	Waist to pelvic portion of the body and organs lying in lower abdominal region
Heel	Pelvic area and sciatic nerve

Inner foot/hand	Half portion of the spine of the right side and half portion of the spin on the left side
Outer area of foot/hand	Arm, shoulder, hip, leg, knee, and lower back
Ankle area of feet/ wrists	Pelvic area, reproductive organs

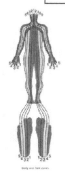

ZONE 1:

Zone 1 starts at the top of the head and runs all the way down to the big toes. It controls everything within that line including:

- Mid forehead
- palate
- lips
- chin
- spine
- abdomen

- legs
- thumb
- shoulders
- arms

The organs that are covered in this zone include:

- head
- brain
- spine
- nose
- mouth
- chin
- pituitary
- pineal
- thyroid
- thymus
- adrenaline
- lungs
- heart
- esophagus
- stomach
- duodenum
- small intestine

- liver

- ureter

- uterus

- sexual organs

- bladder

- rectum

- anus

ZONE 2:

Zone 2 starts at the top of the head, right next to zone one, and runs the entire length of the body, down to the second toe. It also covers down to the very tip of the first finger.

Zone 2 also includes portions of certain organs, including:

- brain

- eyes

- sinuses

- tonsils

- lungs

- bronchial tubes

- heart

- stomach

- liver

- solar plexus

- pancreas

- kidneys

- small intestine

ZONE 3:

Zone three sits directly up against zone 2. It goes from the very top of the head, down to the third toe. It also covers the arm down to the second finger. Pressure points in this zone also control parts of the:

- brain

- eyes

- lungs

- heart

- stomach

- solar plexus

- pancreas

- liver

- kidneys

- appendix

- small intestine

ZONE 4:

Zone 4 starts at the very top of the head and goes all the way down to the fourth toe. It also covers a stretch of the arm, down to the third finger on the hand.

Certain portions of internal organs are covered in this zone as well, including:

- brain

- ears

- shoulders

- lungs

- heart

- stomach

- spleen

- pancreas

- liver

- gallbladder

- appendix

- small intestines

- colon

ZONE 5:

Zone 5, again starts at the very top of the head and goes all the way down to the little toes. It also covers a stretch of the arm on the exterior side that goes down to the tip of the little finger.

Zone 5 also controls portions of some internal organs, including:

- brain

- ears

- shoulders

- upper arms

- spleen

- liver
- gallbladder
- ileocecal valve
- appendix
- colon

FACIAL REFLEXOLOGY

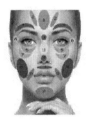

Reflexology also works on various zones of the face. The picture above shows the various centers of the face that can be used to treat different ailments. The information below will help you learn to use these points. The pressure used must be applied using the thumb or finger. The pressure must be gentle, but it also must be deep. In order to achieve the desired result, you must apply pressure for up to seven seconds, and it must be done three times in a row, with a ten second break between pressure applications.

- Menstrual Problems – Apply pressure to area 1
- Head Cold – Apply pressure to areas 2, 4, 8, 9,
- Pelvic problems   - Apply pressure to area 3
- Headaches – Apply pressure to area 5
- Migraine – Apply pressure to areas 6
- Sleep disturbances – Apply pressure to areas 7

- Symptoms associated with menopause – Apply pressure to area 10

- Problems with the throat, cough or asthma symptoms – Apply pressure to area 11

- Toothache (any tooth) - Apply pressure to area 9

- Bed-wetting, urinary discomfort – apply pressure to area 1

- Double vision – apply pressure to area 2

- Insomnia or cold – apply pressure to areas 3 and

- Problems with sciatica, liver, or gallbladder – apply pressure to area 4

- Mental stress – Apply pressure to areas 8 and 10

HOW REFLEXOLOGY WORKS

There has been a lot of study into why reflexology works. While ancient healers did provide a basic guideline on how internal systems and imbalance works, they were very vague in regards to today's standards.

Reflexology essentially clears the body of toxins and things that are considered impurities. These toxins and impurities accumulate on nerves and nerve endings, which ultimately leads to many different problems in the body, one of them being pain. The build up disrupts the normal flow of energy and the ability for nerves to properly conduct information to the brain.

Reflexology helps to break down these deposits. Once the deposits have been broken down through pressure, it is flushed from the body through natural methods.

After reflexology has been completed, it is important that the person it was done on drinks at least 8 glasses of water during the next 24 hour period.

RECOMMENDED DURATION OF REFLEXOLOGY

Each age range has a recommended duration per sitting for reflexology. While reflexology can be done multiple times over a 24 hour period, the length of time per setting should be limited for the patient's sake.

- Newborn to 3 months - No longer than 3 minutes per setting

- 3 months – 6 months – No longer than 4 minutes

- 6 months to 1 year – No longer than 5 minutes

- Children age 1 year to 3 years – No longer than 7 minutes

- Children age 3 years to 12 years – No longer than 10 minutes

- Children 12 years to Adult – No longer than 15 minutes

When you are treating a specific illness, you should not make it a practice to treat those particular areas of the body. You must have a thorough understanding of how parts of the body are related and treat those areas as well.

THE HEART

When the purpose of a reflexologist is to focus on a problem surrounding the heart, they must also focus on contributing factors as well. A reflexology must treat a person holistically since the cardiovascular system is made up of the heart, the arteries, the veins, the arterioles, the venules and the capillaries. Even though the heart is the diagnosed problem, this may not be the exact area the problem is.

The aim of reflexology is to improve circulation and the overall system in a manner that is not invasive, like medication or surgery. After treating the heart, the kidneys are addressed, followed by the diaphragm and the lungs. After the lungs have been treated, the spinal area is treated to ensure a complete openness of the cardiovascular system.

There are times where doctors use a form of reflexology during an actual heart attack while medication is being administered. This helps to reduce the damage that is being done to the heart and the muscles around it.

THE KIDNEYS

The kidneys are an essential part of the process necessary to remove waste from the human body. They collect toxin that have been built up in the circulatory system as the blood passes around the body. Reflexology can help the body to release these toxins from the kidneys and flush them from the body.

ABOUT THE KIDNEYS AND TOXINS

The kidneys should be treated to relieve toxins on a regular basis, especially if someone sees a reflexologist on a regular basis. Not only is it recommended for the sake of keeping toxins out of your body, it is also recommended to prevent serious medical conditions later on down the line. It also helps prevent toxins from building up to the point where they release back into the blood stream, causing further problems that may require medical intervention.

REFLEXOLOGY MAPS

As you know, reflexology makes use of maps that showcase the different pressure points that lie beneath the feet. These maps were all created a long time back and trace its roots to ancient china. The Chinese masters were some of the first ones to create the maps mentioning the different pressure points that lie under the feet. The same maps have been passed down from generation to generation and are now widely used by those that provide reflexology massages. It is interesting to know that these maps are not universal and they differ from master to master. So, you will not have two maps that look the same and each therapist will use a unique and individual technique to stimulate the different internal organs. These maps not only showcase the individual zones that lie in the body but also mention the different pressure points. A layman might not be able to identify the different zones under the feet just by making loose connections. It is important to thoroughly understand which organ is connected to which pressure point under the foot.

REFLEXOLOGY POINTS

As was mentioned earlier, the maps carry the pressure points of the body's organs. You will have the chance to know which pressure point corresponds to what internal organ. As a rule of thumb, all pressure points present under the left foot correspond with the organs that are present on the left side of the body. So if you are looking to stimulate the pancreas or the heart, then their corresponding points will be present under the left foot. Similarly, all the organs that lie on the right side of your body will find their pressure points under your right foot. So, depending on what organ you wish to stimulate, you will be able to apply pressure to the corresponding point that lies under the respective foot. Remember that they will not correspond to the individual points alone and will also connect with the different blood vessels and glands that the organ is connected with.

REFLEXOLOGY TECHNIQUES

There are different reflexology methods that are practiced and you can make use of any technique to avail relief from your conditions.

The Ingham method

The first method is known as the Ingham method. This method is attributed to Eunice Ingham, who is said to have significantly influenced the practice of reflexology. The method is simple to apply and thus makes it one of the most preferred techniques. It calls for people to walk their thumbs over the healing area and apply a consistent pressure. The thumbs both falls flat and create an angle thereby alternating the pressure that stimulates the chosen area. This technique is mostly used to help the patient relax and does not really focus on any one type of internal issue.

SPECIALIZED TECHNIQUES

Apart from these techniques, there are also certain specialized techniques that people use. These are invented based on what the patients wish to avail from the massage. There is no definite technique that people follow and it is mostly devised on the spot.

Rwo Shur method

The Rwo Shur method is another reflexology technique that you can try. It is one of the most widely used techniques in Asia. It involves stimulating the pressure points by pressing on the down on the points and also sliding the thumbs on the area.

Meridian Reflexology

Meridian Reflexology is based on the Traditional Chinese Medicine (TCM) and also Japanese Zen Shiatsu technique to health and wellness.

In Meridian Reflexology, the reflexologist fixes inequalities in the body's power tract by working on the meridian lines on the feet, not the common foot reflexes. The Meridian Reflexology strategy complies with the timeless method to Reflexology because the feet are viewed as mirroring the entire body.

Meridian Reflexology utilizes the Traditional Chinese Medicine (TCM) principle of meridian power paths in the body. These are likewise stood for on the feet. The five aspects of the Chinese technique are Earth, Water, Fire, Metal as well as Wood.

There are 12 'timeless' meridians in the body, which additionally have stations on the feet (based on the Zen Shiatsu method of Shizuto Masunaga). All of the meridians are connected with each other as if to a 'network' via the body and also power or 'chi' is stated to stream with them.

By working with the components of the meridians located on the feet, the reflexologist intends to rebalance the entire body.

Meridian Reflexology is a total therapy by itself, yet I normally have Meridian Reflexology in combo with Precision Reflexology. I deal with particular meridians, as well as acupressure factors.

Ayurveda Reflexology

Eastern and Western philosophies have created special blends to create a reflexology technique called Ayurvedic, which derives from the principles of Ayurveda. It allows therapists to approach the foot and hand work with exciting and unique methods. An Australian woman by the name of Sharon Stathis is a brilliant lady who created this technique. It is now being used in fifteen countries on a routine basis.

What is the main focus of the approach? It is to assist with the energy systems within the body, which could help relax the nervous system, muscle system, cardiovascular system, endocrine system, and much more. A vital flow of energy which is referred to prana. It flows within channels that are micro and are called nadis. If prana and its flow are disturbed in any shape or form; it affects not only the body but the mind as well. This can cause pains throughout the body, muscle cramps, headaches, spasms, body pain as well as controllable thinking. Within these flows, there are points called marma. These are vital energy centers that run along the nadis. The body and it is beneficial when the points are being worked during a reflexology session.

Only oil should be used when working the marma. Unwanted friction is and can cause the delicate energy to be thrown off balance. Is there a specific type of oil being used? The answer is yes. Sesame oil which can be found in most super markets is best used when warm to become a sensual lubricant. It is most preferred during a session.

A bronze bowl from India known as a kasa is an exciting new addition to the therapy. It is treated like any other technique in the field. It is rubbed down with oil to create a warm, sensation against the palms or the soles of the feet. It usually lasts up to five minutes but no less than three. Clients have raved about the wonderful feeling they receive.

The Ayurvedic Reflexology is a different technique being used instead of the norm of massage therapy. It has been known to be a much simpler and gentler approach. It allows the clients body to become relaxed beneath the hands of a practitioner. A 40-45-minute session isn't like any other therapy; it is like the moment of reaching pure desire. Hands and feet are being worked on in conjunction with each other. No client has left unhappy.

These are some of the most widely used reflexology techniques that are used.

HOW DOES REFLEXOLOGY RELATE TO OTHER THERAPIES?

Acupuncture and acupressure is in relation to a reflexology therapy session. These other therapy sessions are able to stimulate the points of the body, which work together to help the other parts. The outcome is the same. They are all trying to achieve the energy flow and bring it a high point of relaxation.

The points in reflexology are the not always the same points used in acupuncture and/or acupressure. There are so many more points that can be used outside of reflexology.

Massage allows the body to relax and reach a point of manipulation of tissues in the body. However, there are specific techniques being used such as tapping or kneading. This is to relax any tension out of the muscles.

These types of therapists are not working from the inside out. But yet they are working from the outside in. This allows the body to be healed before the inner is healed. When a massage is being performed, the client removes clothing, but in reflexology this only occurs on the specific body part being worked on.

A reflexology therapist likes to help the client by stimulating their nervous system to release tension, which is why they are referred to working from the inside out.

ARE THERE TIMES WHEN I SHOULDN'T HAVE REFLEXOLOGY?

There are no real life dangers during a reflexology session. It is safe and very healing to a client. However, a therapist needs to be aware of some things before a session can begin. For example, foot fractures, gout and unhealed wounds should be avoided. These conditions can cause more pain to a client and will help to create a relaxing session.

If the foot cannot be part of the session, then the client has alternative areas to work on such as the ears or hands. However, the same precautions taken with the foot should be taken into consideration. The best interest of the client should come first before any session begins.

Women who are pregnant can have reflexology session but it needs to be altered by using the reflex points in the uterine and ovarian. This can either be done with gentle motions or being avoided altogether.

Children can find great benefits from any of these techniques are found to not have enough patience to last an entire session. Their attention span is not all there.

An overload to your system can occur if you are performing any type of massage therapy or other therapies should be not taken so close together. At least two days should be done in between sessions.

No practitioner will allow a client to be worked on if they have any type of injuries. Gloves will be used if the treated areas are to be compromised.

CHAPTER 3

REFLEXOLOGY BENEFITS

Reflexology has many benefits. Let us look at some of them in this chapter.

REFLEXOLOGY - COMPLEMENTARY AND ALTERNATIVE MEDICINE

Have you ever seen a bottle of herbal medicine at the drugstore and had a curiosity as to whether it would help you fight off that cold? Maybe you have thought about seeing a chiropractor to treat your back pain, instead of swallowing that handful of pills. If this is the case, you are not alone. Every year, there are millions of people who try some type of complementary or alternative medicine. Complementary or alternative medicine typically accompanies the treatment that you are already getting from your family doctor.

Even though so many people try these alternative treatments, you may still wonder if they work. Whether you are wasting your money, whether the remedies are safe? While traditional medicine has begun researching these various treatments, there is a lot more research needed to determine how effective each type of treatment is.

WHAT IS COMPLEMENTARY AND ALTERNATIVE MEDICINE?

These treatments are ones that are not used by most doctors and are not considered "conventional medicine." They consist of a group of practices that have been around for thousands of years, but are still outside the scope of mainstream medicine.

When used alongside mainstream medicine, these treatments are considered complementary. When used instead of mainstream medicine, they are considered alternative medicine. A simple example of using them as a complementary medicine is using Tylenol from the pharmacy, and receiving acupuncture. An example of using them as alternative medicine would be receiving acupuncture, but not taking pain medication.

WHO USES COMPLEMENTARY AND ALTERNATIVE MEDICINE

Research proves that more than 40% of women in the United States alone use complementary and alternative medicine. If you include prayer as a form of complementary medicine, the percentage rises to nearly 69%.

COMPLEMENTARY AND ALTERNATIVE MEDICINE IS USED BY:

- Women
- Men
- People with advanced educational
- Doctors
- Pharmacists

OTHER PEOPLE WHO USE COMPLEMENTARY AND ALTERNATIVE MEDICINE INCLUDE:

- People who conventional medicine has not helped
- People who believe that natural products are healthier than manufactured products
- People who want to add it to their medical regimen to create a holistic experience

SOME OF THE DOWNSIDES OF USING COMPLEMENTARY AND ALTERNATIVE MEDICINE ARE:

- Some forms have not been proven to work
- Some have not been researched enough

- Some are mistakenly thought safe because they are natural, and have turned out to be dangerous, for example: ephedra.

- Some can interfere with the way prescription drugs work

- Some are unsafe during pregnancy

- Some may carry risks that are not known to modern medicine

If you do choose to use a complementary or alternative medicine, you should let your doctor know before starting it. You should ask what their experience has been with patients using the specific treatment you are considering, and whether it is safe with your current medication regimen and therapies.

REFLEXOLOGY/AYURVEDA

Typically, when a type of reflexology is recommended by a doctor, they recommend Ayurveda. This is because Ayurveda combines herbal medicines, meditation and yoga together to help a patient feel more internally balanced. There has been a lot of research done on reflexology and its benefits to the body, but the most positive reports have come from Ayurveda based reflexology.

AYURVEDA

Ayurveda is a system of holistic healing. It is expected to be simple and contain ingredients that cure everyday ailments.

- Neem – Purifies the blood

- Tulsi/Basil – Antiseptic

- Amla/Gooseberry – the purest form of vitamin C that can be foundation

- Brahmi – relieves anxiety, enhances memory, helps with nervous disorders.

- Aloe Vera – used to treat liver and spleen disorders, helps regulate menstruation

- Eucalyptus – helps treat stuffed nose and sore throat, treats acne

- Five-Leaved Chaste – Treats acne, boils, eczema and hair loss

- Sesame – promotes hair growth

- Turmeric – antiseptic

- Karpoor – camphor powder – skin vitalizer

- Virang – treats skin infections

- Indian Barberry – antiseptic

- Coriander – treats digestive disorders, relieves flatulence, helps produce urine, decreases fever

- Chirayata – fever reducer

- Nutmeg – helps treat digestive problems, dehydration, skin disorders, and insomnia.

- Ashoka – Used for reducing menstrual flow

- Sarpagandha – lowers blood pressure

- Peepal – Helps treat heart disease

- Onion – promotes release of toxins from the body

- Kaith – Aromatic to help relieve congestion

- Methi – Treats bad breath

- Clove – relieves flatulence and reduces asthma symptoms

- Bael Fruit – treats constipation, diarrhea, dysentery

- … and there are thousands more!

NERVOUS SYSTEM

The first and foremost importance of reflexology is strengthening the nervous system. It helps in clearing up the neural pathways that makes it easy for the person to experience the different sensations. Brain function will automatically improve and the person will feel much better and lighter after a session.

STRESS/TENSIONS

Reflexology is known to help with the release of stress and anxiety. In fact, most patients avail the treatments for this particular reason alone. They will find it easy to avail relief from their stress, tensions, anxiety and depression. The reflexologist will know which particular pressure points to stimulate in order to help the person get rid of their mental issues. It is possible to cut down on the cortisol and increase the serotonin in the body through reflexology.

ENERGY

You can maintain your energy levels by taking up reflexology. For all those that have reduced energy levels, reflexology will not only increase your energy but will also assist in controlling adrenaline function. So, you will have the right amount of energy at all times.

DIGESTION

Reflexology can be used to increase digestion and overall digestive power. As you know, it is possible to reach the gut, intestines and stomach regions of the body through the different corresponding points and it will go a long way in helping you improve your digestive capacity.

IMMUNITY

You can improve your immunity to a large extent by taking up reflexology. You can fight away many illnesses by taking up reflexology. It is possible to stimulate your liver where most of the defense mechanism takes place. With better immunity, you will be able to lead a better life.

BLOOD CIRCULATION

It is possible for your body to circulate blood in a better way thanks to reflexology. Reflexology helps in eliminating the different toxins that build up in your body and this can help you maintain healthy and clean blood. The blood vessels are also stimulated and invigorated and you will feel quite healthy after a session.

HEADACHES/ MIGRAINES

You can beat headaches and migraines thanks to reflexology. If you suffer from headaches often then reflexology will help reduce it to a large extent. Of course it is not possible to completely eliminate it and you will always feel a little pain every once in a while. But you can reduce both the occurrence and the sensation of pain by taking up reflexology.

ENDOCRINE SYSTEM

Reflexology can also help the endocrine system. The endocrine system controls a lot of body activities including hormone production and also keeping the body in balance. Undertaking stress can cause the endocrine system to dysfunction and it becomes all the more important for people to take care of it. One great way is by making use of reflexology. You can speak with your physician about the same.

GRAVE ILLNESSES

It is known that reflexology helps in reliving some of the side effects of grave illnesses such as cancer and heart disease. It was found that such patients experienced less pain, nausea and other such side effects. It also effectively helps in reducing stress and anxiety.

PREGNANCY

Pregnant women experience a lot of side effects such as the swelling of feet, tiredness, nausea etc. With the help of reflexology, it is possible to beat all of these side effects and improve overall health. It is advised that these women get the treatments every once in a while and inform the therapist about the same. They will be able to help the women reduce their pain and discomfort.

INSOMNIA

Those that suffer from insomnia or find it difficult to fall asleep will find it easy to beat both by taking up reflexology. Reflexology helps in inducing sleep as it gets over stress and anxiety. It also stimulates the different pressure points under feet, which aids in improving blood circulation and also assists in the elimination of built up toxins and other unnecessary elements from the body.

KIDNEY ISSUES

You can also avail some relief from kidney issues. Reflexology has the capacity of reaching nearly all the organs inside the body. You can consult with your reflexologist and ask them about the massages that will help with kidney issues.

SINUS

Those suffering from sinus problems can avail a lot of relief from their sinus issues. Sinus causes people respiratory issues and also pain in the forehead and upper cheeks. This can be easily dealt with by using reflexology. The therapist will know which areas under the feet to stimulate in order to eliminate any sinus issues.

Remember that you have to undertake regular sessions in order to experience these positive benefits. Undertaking it every once in a while will not work for you. You have to indulge in it at least twice a month and more is always good. If you suffer from any condition, then you have to first speak with your doctor before taking up any of the treatments.

STEP INTO PROPER CARE OF YOUR FEET

Taking excellent care of your feet is of prime importance. Your feet take a beating every day, and as your body's foundation, they carry you wherever you go. Therefore, it is a wise plan to stay tuned to their daily needs.

A human foot, with its incredible weight-bearing capabilities has 25 bones, 30 joints, and 100 muscles, tendons, and ligaments. This gives them flexibility and strength which enables them to perform their monumental task.

Preventive maintenance and care cannot be stressed enough and each of our expertly-trained medical professionals are there to keep your feet in top shape. This way if any problems may happen to come up with your feet, especially as we age, our trained staff will be ready to make all the difference.

Your feet are not shy in telling you specifically where any extra pressure problems may be located and if your shoes are causing any inflammation or callous build-up. Seeing to these problems will benefit your comfort levels while walking while also improving the foot condition in itself. Having ill-fitted shoes can have a great effect on the health of your feet.

Main Benefits of Foot Care

· Keeping nails trim and clean will help avoid and control ingrown nails and stop any infection that may set in.

· Getting rid of unnecessary excess skin build-up will help reduce the pain and discomfort of corns, callouses and bunions.

· Enjoying the relaxation of a foot massage not only benefits your well-worked feet, it also helps with circulation and sends beneficial nerve impulses and energy to all other parts of the body that may need it. And your feet will really appreciate it after a hard day's work.

· Stress levels are immediately reduced

Additional Benefits of Foot Care

Regular appointments can really benefit anyone who is suffering from arthritis in their feet. A gentle massage will soothe the feet and as arthritis is benefited by the use of heat, a paraffin wax treatment will send penetrating warmth to those painful joints.

Foot Care and Diabetes

As previously mentioned, special care of the feet is of prime concern for diabetics. Some serious foot conditions may result from the damage to nerves, etc. incurred from high levels of glucose in the blood. It's easy to bypass these problems due to the general foot numbness experienced by many people with diabetes. Therefore, daily vigilance and preventative care is very important. It may be a wise idea to visit a specialist in foot care at least once per month for this purpose.

When to Seek Immediate Care

Be watchful of the condition of your feet. They need to be in top shape to continue with their important job. Contact your foot care specialist if any of the following conditions happen to occur.

· Foot pain or any numbness

- Wounds that won't heal

- Any visible changes in the shape of the foot or toes

- Any unusual conditions

- Benefits of Reflexology for PMS

PMS affects a large percentage of women during their reproductive years. Many of the exasperating symptoms are anxiety, depression, mood swings, bloating, cramping, headaches, etc. It usually will occur approximately two weeks before the onset of menses.

These symptoms range from moderate to severe and often worsen as the person gets closer to menopause in their later years. Treating symptoms with over-the-counter medications often produce unwanted side-effects and is often not the answer. Studies that have been conducted in many different parts of the world have shown that reflexology can help with symptoms of PMS.

Since using Reflexology helps the body return to a condition of homeostasis which is its natural balance within its internal environment. Reflexology helps the body heal by aiding in un-blocking any obstructions and improving energy flow. It focuses on reflex points in the foot that influence particular glands, as well as the ones responsible for reproductive health. It relieves stress and pain, can help with sleep issues, and improve energy. Women have reported improvement with their PMS, sometimes after one session. Everyone will react and improve at a different pace.

Reflexology can help in surprising ways. For example, it can relieve bloating and retaining water by improving the function of both kidneys and bladder by assisting in flushing out excess fluids.

MEDITATION AND REFLEXOLOGY

Concentrating on healing and your body during a reflexology session is a wonderful aid in helping with the flow of energy. Not only should the practitioner concentrate but so should the client so that all positive thought and function goes to improving the success of the session. Some clients will try to picture the energy flowing to improve any problem areas while a session is occurring. This can only help in the positive effect.

SOME CONDITIONS IMPROVED BY REFLEXOLOGY

Reflexology works by improving any blockages and increasing energy flow in the body. A session sends specific nerve impulses throughout the entire body as well as specific physical areas at once. By using the zones of the body and the particular reflexes of the foot a practitioner will focus on helping the body to heal itself. Gentle pressure is used, often relieving painful 'deposits' (which are like gritty bumps) under the skin that directly relate to specific problems in the body.

FOLLOWING ARE JUST SOME OF THE PARTICULAR CONDITIONS THAT HAVE BEEN HELPED BY REFLEXOLOGY

- Shoulder Pain/Back Pain/Neck Pain
- Injuries from Accidents
- Insomnia
- PMS
- Migraines
- Arthritis/Tendonitis/Bursitis

WHAT TO EXPECT DURING A REFLEXOLOGY SESSION

Having a Reflexology session is actually very relaxing and in itself is a stress reliever. The room is often darkened and there may be soft background music. The pressure is fairly light and often relieves a mild pain in that area of the foot that is akin to relieving tight muscles during a massage. It is recommended to wear loose clothes to optimize the relaxing effect of the session. A session will usually take around an hour to complete.

TWO EASY TO DO CHINESE REFLEXOLOGY TECHNIQUES

Chinese has created therapy known as Chinese zone therapy. The zone and points on the feet, hands and ears have been linked to all the body's glands, parts as well as organs. The difference felt after a session with these techniques intact are well worth it.

Not only is the flow of energy being brought back to life but it also brings a cleansing to all the body and its components. It helps to treat illnesses such as headaches.

An introduction to various procedures that can be practiced at home safely and will give you relaxation as well a new found energy to your body.

The ears have more than a hundred points that are active. If you grab entire ear and simply pull on them at least twenty times in all directions, they help to release energy. This will cause a burning sensation which in most cases is a warm pleasant feeling not just in your ears but your entire body as well.

Covering your ears with your palms as if you are plugging them will help circulate the energy to flow. This should be done at up to four times. These techniques can be done either in the morning times or whenever you need a boost of energy.

When applying pressure to the skin with your thumbs, it is best not to use heavy pressure. Light and firm is the key when using reflexology to relax.

The feet are another source of a reflexology point. When trying to release energy from this area, it is best to be in a sitting position such as on a bed or chair and to place a foot on your opposite thigh. This position allows you to give your foot full attention. A gentle massage the bottom of the foot in circular motions will release energy and create a blissful sensation throughout the entire body.

The foot reflexology is basically massaging the area from top to bottom in sensual and circular motion. Feet have points such as other body parts to create bursts of energies. Creams and/or oils of your favorite brand or scents can be used to create a higher reflexology session. Both feet should be treated equal.

No matter which therapy technique you decide to perform, a physician should always be notified, especially when symptoms start to arise when starting anything new. Everybody is different and react according to how their body operates.

CHAPTER 4

SOME TIPS TO BEAR IN MIND

WHILE PRACTICING REFLEXOLOGY

Here are some standard tips that you must bear in mind when you take up reflexology.

DO YOUR RESEARCH

The first tip is to do as much research on the topic as possible. Don't take it up if you are not sure how to go about it. You might end up making mistakes that can hurt the patient. Go through this book again if you like to understand the proper techniques and various benefits of the procedures. Once you are sure you have understood the techniques properly, you can take them up.

COMPLETE THE TREATMENT

Remember to always complete a treatment and not leave it abruptly. When you start stimulating a person's feet, you should do the entire length of the foot right from the toe tips to the base of the feet. You must also massage the person's hands and ears if they require stimulation. If you don't complete the treatment, then the person might not be able to avail benefits of the massage.

ASK ABOUT PRESSURE

If you have ever had a reflexology session, then you would have noticed the reflexologist asking you about the pressure from time to time. This is an important aspect of reflexology and you have to ask the patient from time to whether the pressure you are applying is proper or needs to be increased or decreased.

Remember that everybody's threshold differs and applying the same kind of pressure on all might lead to injury. So ask at the beginning and keep asking throughout the session just to be sure.

POWDER OVER OIL

Many reflexologists use oil or lotion to massage feet. However, it would be a better idea for you to use powder or talc as that will help you have a better grip. If the person already has oily skin and you apply more oil, then it will only make it extremely slippery for you. The fingers or feet slipping away from your grip might cause injury to your patient and it is important that you exercise due precaution. If you really have to use oil, then you can use a non-slippery variety.

FOOT IS BEST

Many people agree that foot reflexology is the best as it provides faster relief from the conditions. Although hand and ear will also work well, they might take some time to show results. You will also find a lot of information on foot reflexology and that will help you perform the techniques with ease. Even if you plan to do hands and ears, you can start with the foot first and then move to hands and ears.

DON'T RUSH

Don't be in a hurry to finish all the treatments. You have to take it slow. Rushing it will only cause you to leave the practice incomplete. Most sessions take around 45 minutes and can be reduced to 30 minutes if needed. You must not be in a hurry to go somewhere, as that will cause you to leave the practice incomplete. Allot enough time for it before taking up the practice and then go through with it. You also need to wait for the person to start moving around after the treatment is done and only then take leave.

TELL PATIENTS ABOUT REFLEXES

You have to know that reflexology generally causes reflexes. These reflexes refer to responses that they body will automatically generate after a session. These reflexes will differ from person to person and so will the degree. In any case, you have to tell your patients in advance about the reflexes that they can expect after a session. Some of the common reflexes include coughing, sneezing, burping and muscle contractions. You should tell your patients to expect these and they are normal reflexes.

SUGAR PATIENTS

You must understand that sugar patients will have a different reaction to reflexology. You have to advise them to check their sugar level before the treatment and also after in order to see if it is normal. Reflexology is known to spike up sugar levels or also considerably reduce it after a session. So it is best to ask your patient to have it checked out in advance.

COMFORT IS A 2-WAY STREET

It is important that the patient be comfortable when you massage his or her feet. You should ask them to lie down on their back and enquire if they are comfortable. You too must be comfortable and find a relaxing pose. If you are not sitting comfortably then it will impact your session and the patient will also feel it. Make sure you are sitting on a low stool that helps you reach the other person's feet with ease.

DON'T FORGET TO SANITIZE

Don't forget to sanitize your hands after massaging someone's feet. It might not be practical to use gloves or wash your hands each time. You can maintain a bottle of sanitizer and use it after each massage session. You have to first apply some sanitizer on the person's feet so that you can get rid of most of the germs on it.

SOAK

It is a good idea to soak the person's feet in warm water first so that the skin softens and you can easily massage. The water should be tepid and not too hot. Ask your patient if the temperature is proper by first dipping in just their toes.

You have to bear these tips in mind every time you wish to perform the massages.

REFLEXOLOGY: LEGITIMATE FORM OF MODERN MEDICINE OR JUST A PASSING FANCY?

Is the Western, alternative form of medicine referred to as reflexology a truly effective, reliable procedure that is helping people across the globe heal life-altering, debilitating illnesses and conditions or is it just a farce being tested on unsuspecting, desperate patients who will try anything to alleviate pain, symptoms, or chronic illnesses?

The word itself almost puts you in mind of a contemporary, trendy, complicated, new-age science. Sort of like something a young scientist came up with in an effort to get all the rich, famous, elite, celebrity types to jump on board, spending wads of cash just to be part of the elite, "It Crowd".

WHAT IS REFLEXOLOGY, HOW LONG HAS IT BEEN IN PRACTICE, AND WHERE DID IT START?

The reality of the assumed lack of knowledge, logic, education, understanding, and acceptance of reflexology, however, is this: It is actually a highly researched, tremendously reliable, completely legitimate form of medical treatment that's basis is formed solely on a sequence of procedures including massage, detoxification, and applying pressure to hands, feet, and heads. Reflexology is an alternative form of medicine proven to be particularly effective and has been used in Eastern civilizations such as China and Japan for thousands of years using techniques such as applying tree roots and extracts to help eliminate numerous ailments.

The system of Reflexology was introduced in the United States in the early 1900s. William H. Fitzgerald, M.D. determined the concept of Reflexology in 1913 while practicing as an ear, nose, and throat specialist. Shortly after William's findings, Dr. Edwin Bowers Fitzgerald established the theory that applying pressure produced a somewhat analgesic, pain-relieving effect. These anesthetic qualities not only relieved the areas where pressure was applied, it miraculously seemed to produce calmative relief in other unrelated areas of the body.

Since its discovery in the beginning of the 20th century in America, as well as around the world, research, practice, testing, and administration of reflexology indicate individuals reporting partial or even complete alleviation of the conditions that the reflexology help was originally sought after. Reflexology has even been said to be responsible for relief of additional, unrelated problems and various conditions. Some uses in particular include using an intervention or interception of sorts to decrease or even eliminate pain, enhance relaxation, reduce stress, detoxify, alleviate urinary symptoms, and reduce and diminish psychological symptoms, such as anxiety and depression.

There are quite a few other benefits and positive results that will ultimately occur when utilizing reflexology simply because the reflex points in the hands, feet, and head are actually directly linked to each and every individual part of the body. This means that the ability to stimulate nerve function is increased, and individual's energy level increases, the circulatory system is more efficient, boosting circulation, it is common for people to have higher immunities and recover quicker from injuries or surgeries, and finally, an individual's behavior, attitude, lifestyle and quality of life can all be immensely improved.

DETOXIFICATION UTILIZED IN INCREASING REFLEXOLOGY EFFECTIVENESS – DOES IT WORK?

So, the big question in regards to this topic is: What is

Detoxification and how does it work? Detoxification is simply the process of cleaning an individual's blood. The process of cleaning an individual's blood involves removing any impurities that travel to the liver in the form of toxins, which are processed for removal in the form of waste. Our bodies naturally rid themselves of some toxins via lungs, intestines, lymph, skin, kidneys, etc., although it is impossible to naturally eliminate ALL toxins. The food we consume, the air we breathe, and a variety of other miscellaneous environmental factors cause toxins to build up in our bodies. The excessive build-up of these impurities can cause ailments such as cardiovascular complications, liver disorders, stomach and intestinal issues, infertility and impaired brain function. A related perk to cleansing and detoxifying is the cleaning up of urinary infections and cleansing of the colon. The efficiency of both the urinary tract and removal of waste through a colon free of toxin build-up is crucial to good health.

Typically, Western medicine tends to rely on surgical procedures, prescription medications, and fad diets. The reason for these chemically induced, temporary fixes is because, as a culture we are lacking the knowledge and understanding that is essential to utilize detoxification effectively. For 1000 years, Chinese and Japanese medical professionals have applied various roots and extracts from trees and tree trunks on humans' bodies. These applications are for the purpose of removing all types of ailments. As a culture, they believe that infections, swelling of body parts and/or organs, congestion, blood flow, chronic and temporary pain and impurities and toxins can literally be extracted from a person by applying a plaster or dressing made of herbs in combination with tree extracts.

Incidentally, recent production of patches designed to remove toxins have become a detoxification tool of choice. The patches are applied to the sole of the foot at night before going to bed and removed in the morning and discarded. When applied, the herbal, self-adhesive patches are clean and white, while, in contrast, when removed they appear visibly dirty. The dirt is

NOT dirt that has come off the foot, but rather toxins and impurities that have been extracted from the body and redistributed to the patch overnight. After a few weeks of use, the patches begin to appear cleaner each morning, signifying fewer toxins present in the body, which would indicate that the patches are working as intended.

It almost seems hard to believe that by simply applying a little pressure to your foot or massage a reflex point in your hand, it can help your entire body. The bottom line, in terms of healing, wellness, effectiveness, and success when treating a human body with reflexology, detoxification, and all the related components is that our bodies have reflex points and when these points are stimulated, triggered, or massaged, the results are tremendous.

CONCERNS AND NEGATIVE REACTIONS TO RESEARCH FINDINGS

Some reviewers of the research, however, feel that the accuracy and possibility of biases due to incomplete or inadequate sampling of patients, doctors, researchers, professionals, etc. in regards to reflexology studies is inconsistent and that much more specific, high-quality, educated research is needed. The downside to this increase in the standards of testing and researching is, of course, a need for more funding, education and training, an increase in several capacities of staff members, and time. After all, it has taken hundreds of years for the Western culture to prove their conclusions regarding the practice of reflexology as an established philosophy formulated on the premise that the different zones and reflex points in an individual's body can link ailments, illnesses, pain, behavior, and quality of life by simply applying pressure to their feet, heads, and hands.

CANCER TREATMENT, DIABETES, MULTIPLE SCLEROSIS, MENOPAUSAL RELATED ANXIETY/DEPRESSION, MIGRAINE/TENSION HEADACHES

Cancer Treatment

Although few studies have been done to this point, there have been findings that link reduction of some pain, nausea, bowel issues, anxiety and depression in addition to a seemingly better quality of life when using reflexology treatment along with other cancer treatments.

Diabetes Type II

When dealing with symptoms of Type II Diabetes, foot and hand tingling is often a prevalent side effect. By administering foot reflexology on your own feet or massage reflex points in your own hands, it is believed there could be positive effects, although the inadequacy in clinical outcomes reporting and the lack of consistent numbers of studies may obscure the results.

Multiple Sclerosis

The American Academy of Neurology has been said to be exploring possible alternative medication for individuals with multiple sclerosis. To date, there are un-confirmed presumptions that reflexology is somewhat effective in reducing tingling but only Level C evidence.

Post-Menopausal Related Anxiety and Depression

In a small-sampled study recorded by Williamson et al (2002) the presumption was made that reflexology and foot massage were both helpful in preventing or reducing anxiety and depression in post-menopausal women.

Migraine/Tension Headache

There have been random sampling tests done on patients experiencing migraine or tension related headaches. After a session utilizing foot reflexology, as well as at another 3-month follow-up, the results of several of the patients showed that foot reflexology closely as effective as drug therapy.

CHAPTER 5

TYPES OF REFLEXOLOGY

There are three main types of reflexologies and they are foot reflexology, hand reflexology and ear reflexology.

FOOT REFLEXOLOGY

Foot reflexology is the most common type of reflexology that is practiced around the world.

Foot reflexology is a technique where the therapist massages under the feet and reaches the internal organs of the body. As you know, you have to map out the individual places under the feet to know which organ corresponds to what area below the foot.

You have to refer to a chart for the same. As a general rule, all organs that lie on the right side of the body are available under the right foot and all organs on the left side are under the left foot.

You have to understand the different zones in order to know how to stimulate them.

There are a whole host of benefits that can be availed through foot reflexology including blood circulation, stress removal and bringing in a balance in the body.

The most common massage technique used in foot reflexology is "thumb" walking. Here is how you can perform it.

- Start by observing the tops of your thumbs

- Now place them next to each other so that the sides of the nails just about touch

- Now, see the part where the thumbs touch each other

- That is the part you will be using to walk over the person's feet

- The next step is for you to train your thumb for the massage routine

- Find an object or instrument that can easily slide in between your thumbs

- Most people prefer to hold a pen as it is quite comfortable

- Now hold the pen in your hand

- With your free hand, place the part of the thumb that you will use to massage over the pen

- Now start bending and straightening your thumb without the pen moving

- You should notice the pen moving down from your hand and also the pressure applied by your thumb on the pen increasing

- You have to keep this practice going until your thumb starts to bend and unbend through out

- Once you think you have perfected the motion, you should try the action on your other hand

- You can also practice it on a flat and smooth surface like a table or against the wall

RELAXING MASSAGE

- Start by placing the person's foot on your thighs and make them comfortable

- You have to loosen the person's feet a little by

shaking the feet and then wringing the toes

·   Now hold the tops of their toes with one hand and the bottom of their foot in your other hand

·   You have to now massage the spinal area of the foot

·   These refer to the lines that run down the entire length of the feet on either side and also the area that lies just below the big toe

·   Stimulating this region helps in relieving a lot of stress and pain

·   You have to twist your fingers away from the area so that the person feels a slight pinch

·   When you twist away, you must keep it there for a few seconds each

·   You have to keep walking the thumb back up and down low to stimulate the area as best as you can

·   This will leave the person feeling completely relaxed and also stimulate their spine

TOE ROTATIONS

·   Rotating the toes is a great exercise and will leave the patient feel calm and relaxed

·   For this, start by holding the tops of the toes and rotate it in the clockwise direction first and then anti-clockwise

·   You have to hold the tops firmly so that the bottoms also rotate well

·   Next, hold the part of the toe that lies just above the joint and twist it around

·   Now twist and rotate the bottoms of the toes at the

joints

· These types of twists and turns of feet greatly help in increasing the flow of blood to the head and nourishes the mind

MERIDIAN STIMULATION

· Next, you should stimulate the meridian points in your feet

· These lie just under the nail of each toe except the middle toe

· You have to use the tips of your thumbs to apply a balanced pressure under the nail of each toe

· You can choose both a clock wise and an anti-clockwise motion on each toe

· You have to maintain the motion on each of the toes for 25 to 30 seconds each

THUMB WALKING THE TOES

· Next, you have to thumb walk the toes

· Start at the base of each toe and then make your way to the top or tip

· Keep this motion going for the next 15 to 20 minutes

· Remember that the pressure you apply to the toes differs for each one and you must try and ask them every few minutes about the pressure you are applying

STIMULATING THE CHEST

· The ball of the foot that is located just under the big toe corresponds with the chest area of the body

- You can walk your thumb over this area in order to stimulate and invigorate the chest area

- Be a little gentle while invigorating this area

- You can the thumb walk from the toes to the back of the foot

- The back region can be quite sensitive and the reflexes that people experience when this part is stimulated can be a bit on the higher side

- People will feel tickled and other such sensations when stimulated

STIMULATING THE STOMACH

- Next, you have to stimulate the stomach area of the person

- This area is represented by the thinnest area under the foot and varies from person to person

- You can locate the area by rubbing under the foot and then finding the thinnest area

STIMULATING THE PELVIC REGION

- It is important to stimulate the pelvic region, especially for women

- You can find the exact location by looking at the chart and finding the right area

- The right area is located over the sciatic nerve and by stimulating it, you can reach the pelvic region

- From the thinnest part, walk your thumbs back to the back of the feet

STIMULATING GUT AND INTESTINES

- You can stimulate the gut and intestines by finding the right area below the foot

- You have to use a particular angle to massage under the feet in order to alleviate the pain

Once done, you have to offer the person water to drink or also green tea. You must ask them to remain hydrated in order to avail maximum benefit of the massage therapy.

HAND REFLEXOLOGY

As you know, the human brain is closely connected to the different reflexes. However, what most people don't realize is that any reflex action that occurs is mostly a result of an automatic impulse and the brain is not giving it any directions to do so. The brain will then feel the pain of the activity and react to it in a different way.

With the use of hand reflexology, you will be able to influence the reflex action time.

With hand reflexology, you will make use of the same technique as you would with your foot reflexology. However, you must know that the pressure points on your hands will be much more deep seated and you have to apply a little extra pressure while trying to reach them. You will know to apply the appropriate pressure when you start massaging.

RELAXING MASSAGE

- To massage the hands, start by twisting the wrists and then push the thumb upwards

- Create simple circular motions on the palm for 25 to 30 seconds

- Once the front of the hand is done, you can move to the back of the hand

·   You can start by stimulating the knuckles and then push the fingers towards the wrist

·   Keep enquiring about the pressure to make sure that they are comfortable

·   Now lightly squeeze individual fingers and move them from side to side

·   You can move them from right to left and left to right in sequence

·   The joints at the fingers need to feel pliable and increase the lubrication at the joints

·   Press gently the wrists and shake the hand from side to side

STIMULATING THE MERIDIANS

·   The meridians on the fingers are all located at different points

·   To stimulate them, you must find the exact locations and apply equal pressure on them to affect the different areas

·   The main areas that get affected by the stimulation include the heart area, the lungs and the intestines

·   You have to finish the massage by stimulating the points by turning them both clockwise and anti-clockwise

STIMULATING THE FINGERS

·   The fingers are connected to a large number of organs inside the body

·   You can influence many blood vessels, organs and muscles by stimulating the fingers

- As is with the toes, you must start from the top of the fingers and then make your way down slowly to the base of the fingers

- You have to stimulate the fingers from top to base by applying equal pressure

STIMULATING THE TORSO

- The palm of the hand represents the torso of a person

- By stimulating the center, you will work towards invigorating the liver, gut, intestines and stomach region

- As you know, the center is always lighter in color and the top and sides are dark

- Each one stands for a different internal organ and pressing them will help you invigorate a different region

- You must always start with the spongy part that is located under the fingers

- Apply light and equal pressure

- Now move towards the outer rim of the palms

- You have to get the person to place their hands on a flat surface and can place it on your lap

- Now work on the thumb

- You have to start from the bottom and then move to the tip of the thumb

- Once done, you must shake the hands

STIMULATING THE BACK OF THE HAND

- The back of the hand holds equal importance and you should work on it just as you would with the front

- The back of the hand has a lot of veins that are prominent which makes it a highly sensitive region of the hand

- To stimulate it, you must be a little gentle and press it lightly

- You must avoid being too hard and keep asking if the person is comfortable

- Start from the knuckle region and the move towards the base of the palms

- Apply pressure all over the wrists and hand and turn and twist the hands to remove any tensions that might exist there

- You can then repeat the same process on the left hand

- It is understood that a person's dominant hand is generally less sensitive as compared to the other one, so, you might have to ask them about the pressure several times before going ahead with the massage

- Once done, hold both hands together and shake it to create ripples

- Offer the patient water to drink or green tea if they prefer it

EAR REFLEXOLOGY

Ear reflexology is the newest form of reflexology that is gaining popularity. It deals with stimulating the ears to reach the different organs of the body. It is believed that the ears are some of the most sensitive regions of the body and by stimulating it, you can invigorate a person.

The basic principle works on stimulating the central nervous system of CNS. This is an important part of the body and you can control a large part of your mind and body by stimulating it.

According to traditional Chinese practitioners, there are around 91 auricular points that are connected to the ear and you can stimulate them by massaging the ear. You can understand where each of these points lie on the ear based on a chart that you can download from the Internet.

Ear reflexology has gained much popularity in the last few years owing to its tendency in reducing pain almost instantly. You will feel much better and fitter after taking up ear reflexology and the results will last you a while. However, it is important for you to consult a bona fide practitioner if you wish to avail lasting benefits. They will tell you where lies the problem and will also tell you what needs to be stimulated in order to help you feel better.

Let us now look at how you can perform ear reflexology on a patient

- As you know, the very first step is to ask if the person is comfortable

- You must also sit in a comfortable position

- You must look at a chart in advance to know where the different points lie on your ear and what they are individually connected to

- You can make use of a hair band for men to prevent their hair from interfering with the massage and women's hair should be tied in a pony tail

- The first thing to stimulate is the ear lobes. Start by gently pulling it down and causing the ear lobes to stretch

- That will get the blood flowing in the ears

- Now use gentle motion to trace the outer region of the ears

· You must invigorate all the senses that are connected to this region and try to stop at every pressure point

· Enquire about the pressure and adjust it accordingly

· It is important that you know what exactly you are stimulating if you wish to prevent any injuries from taking place

· Remember to always have gentle hands and not put too much pressure

· It is best to always work on the outer ear first and then move the fingers inwards

· If the patient is complaining about pain, then you must see which area is aching

· Once you locate it, you can gently press over it to see if the pain subsides

· Once you are done with the outside of the ear, you can make use of a small blunt stick to invigorate the points that lie inside the ear and help your patient avail relief

· Once done, you can pull the tops of the ear a few times

· Offer the patient some water and then ask them to relax a bit

CHAPTER 6

REFLEXOLOGY AND BODY BALANCE

You can make use of reflexology to attain body balance. Body balance refers to aligning the body parts in such a way that it helps in centering the body.

Here is how you can balance the body.

LEG BALANCE

- Leg balance is done to check if the person's legs are in balance with their body

- As you know, sometimes, it becomes important for people to balance their bodies which might change in balance owing to many reasons such as physical and mental reasons

- The first step is to make the person lie down in front of you on a completely flat surface

- It is best to pick something like the floor

- Now get them to raise their hands above their head and bend it backwards

- Now use a pen to mark the topmost point of the ankle bones on either legs

- Now ask the person to place their hands by their sides and sleep normally

- Now join their ankles and see if the two legs match correctly

- If they do, then the person's legs are in perfect

balance, if they don't match then the person's legs are not in balance

- You will have to fix this issue

- Start by looking for the short leg amongst the two

- The ankle point of this leg will lie a little above the other ankle

- To fix this issue, start by placing a firm hand on the knee and then push the ankles backwards towards the body of the person

- Ask if the person is comfortable and if they are in pain then stop the practice immediately

- Now check to see if it has aligned properly

- If not, keep pushing it a little back

- Once done, ask the person to take a walk

- If you wish to use the long leg to fix the issue, then you can lift it up and keep pushing it backwards

- The leg to pick will depend on the person's level of pain, ask them which leg hurts and choose the other one to balance

HIP BALANCE

- To balance the hips, start by making your patient lie down on the left side

- Now use your thumb to place over the middle of their butt and press it down firmly

- Ask them if they are comfortable and if they experienced any difference in their hip joint

- If your patient is slightly heavy, then the above method might not be effective with them

- You will have to press on a spot on the elbow area as that will help you access the joints much easily

- Now ask your patient to flip to the right side and perform the same steps as above

BACK BALANCE

- The next step is to balance the back

- Get the patient to lie on their stomach

- Now lift their head, neck and spine and lift it backwards

- You have to now identify the two distinct dimples that are present on the lower back

- Once you do, you can place your thumbs on the dimples and twist and turn it around to fix the issue in the back

- Now stimulate the spine by pushing your fingers up and down to stimulate the lower back

- Ask if the person is experiencing any pain or discomfort

SOLAR PLEXUS

- The next step is to massage the solar plexus

- They are many vital nerves that lie just behind the stomach region

- Make the patient lie in front of you on their back

- Now check if they have an imbalance in their plexus

region or just check their pulse by checking it on the wrist region

·   If their toes are not aligning properly then it means, there is an imbalance

·   Now lift their legs up in the air and refrain from bending the knees

·   Ask if the person is experiencing any pain

·   Now slowly bring the leg back down to the floor

·   You must repeat this step around 10 to 12 times

·   For a faster result you can also pull the shorter toe outwards until balance is restored

·   Again, keep asking if your patient is comfortable

·   In an alternate procedure, you can place a small cup over the navel area of the person and create a mini vacuum to around it

·   Now you have to wait until such time as the vacuum automatically releases without you tampering with it

SHOULDER BALANCE

·   Tie the person's hair up so that the neck area appears clearly

·   Start by locating the triangle shape that lies on the back of the neck

·   Now place your thumb in the center of this area and while pressing it gently, ask your patient to draw in deep breaths

·   Now release the pressure on the person's neck and get them to inhale, exhale deeply

- Do the same around 5 times

- Keep asking if the patient is comfortable

NECK BALANCE

- It is equally important for you to balance the person's neck

- To do so start by making the person lie down on his or her back in a comfortable position

- Now use a twisted or rolled up piece of soft cloth and balance their neck on it

- Now lift gently and start massaging the neck by applying minimal pressure

- Now provide a little traction to the neck such that it causes a movement in the person's toe

- Now maintain the same position for a while and then release it

- Repeat the same 5 or 6 times and keep enquiring if the patient is comfortable

STOMACH BALANCE

- Start by making the patient lied down in front of you

- Now use your index, middle and ring finger to gently press under the rib cage

- The pressure that you apply should be consistent and slightly gentle

- Now place your other thumb over these fingers and press them down firmly

- Now slightly slide your fingers and then move them

up again

- Do the same 3 to 4 times

- Ask whether the person is comfortable

ABDOMEN BALANCE

- Start by making the person lie down in front of you

- Now use your thumb to apply a gentle pressure at the base of the abdomen

- Now move your finger around from one area of the abdomen to the other and keep the pressure evened out

- Repeat the same around 5 to 6 times

- Ask if the patient is comfortable

These form the different steps to follow while trying to balance the body of your patient.

CHAPTER 7

SPORTS REFLEXOLOGY

It is important to note that reflexology has general benefits for the body and also some special ones that particularly cater to athlete's bodies. Here are some sports injuries with which reflexology helps and also how it helps.

INJURIES

Sprains

Sprains are extremely common in the world of sports and refer to the twisting of muscles. Sprains might be common but the pain they bring along can be quite grueling. With the help of reflexology, you will be able to provide quick relief from sprains and strains that might occur in the limbs, knees, ankles, neck, thumbs etc.

Backache

Backaches are also quite common in the sporting world. Right from tennis players to footballers and also baseball players, backache is one of the most common complaints. But with the help of reflexology, you will be able to help people avail relief from their back pain and also induce better blood circulation.

Knee pain

Knee pain is also a common complaint that people have in sports. But with reflexology, you can put an end to it.

Shoulder injuries

Those that play basketball or tennis will suffer from shoulder injuries. They can avail relief from it by implementing reflexology.

Fractures

It is not possible for an athlete to not experience fractures. When a lot of pressure is applied to the body, it is highly possible that bones will be affected by it. And the most common bone injury is a fracture. So, you have to remain prepared for fracture treatments if you wish to provide reflexology help to athletes.

Hamstrings

Hamstrings are muscles that are present behind your legs. They are extremely stiff and trying to straighten them will almost always cause injury. But through reflexology, you will be able to massage and loosen them and help prevent injuries. You can also affect the pressure points and further strengthen them.

Inflammations

Inflammations are quite common with sports injuries. Rubbing the muscles the wrong way might cause them to flare up and this can cause extreme pain. Through the application of reflexology, you will be able to reduce this inflammation to a large extent.

Joint aches

Joint aches will almost always arise especially if there is repetitive movement involved such as moving of rackets or swinging a cricket bat. With the help of reflexology, you will be able to deal with these aches and pains.

Ankle twists

Ankle twists mainly occur when you partake in sports that require you to run fast and make sharp movements with your feet. With reflexology, you can easily deal with these injuries.

WHY IT HELPS

The first and obvious use of reflexology in the world of sports is to provide quick relief from injuries. As you know, it is possible for a person to maintain a fit and healthy body by reducing the effects of injuries that he or she acquires through paying physical sports.

The next benefit is that, reflexology helps in draining the lactic acid from the body thereby decreasing the stiffness. This lactic acid builds over time and is what can cause catches. But through regular implementation of reflexology, you will be able to put an end to such issues.

Reflexology also helps in increasing the blood circulation to the area that is affected by injury. As you know, blood is full of nutrients and carries fresh oxygen to the different parts of the body. When the affected area is nourished with fresh blood, it helps in increasing the body's capacity to heal and accentuates the healing process.

When an athlete performs the same kind of activity repeatedly for a long period of time, the area that undertakes the most activity starts to develop a consistent pain. Such pain is generally reduced through surgery where the part is operated. However, with the help of reflexology, you will be able to avoid the need for any surgery. The practice alone will help in reducing the pain and inflammation and you will be able to return back to normalcy after a while.

One great aspect of reflexology is that it does not come with any side effects. You can easily implement it and avail relief from your sports injuries.

CHAPTER 8

GETTING A DEGREE AND STARTING

YOUR BUSINESS

If you are confident about your practice and have had rave reviews from people who have availed your service, then you can consider starting your own center.

If you don't know how to go about it, then here is a step-by-step procedure that you can follow.

ATTEND A COURSE

This book will help you get started with reflexology no doubt. But, in order to open a center, you will need a bona fide degree that you can get by attending a course. You can look up a college or any reliable center that provides you both training and will give you a certificate of authenticity. There might be a test that you might have to pass at the beginning in order to attend the course. Once you do, you have to check out the fee structure. Once you settle everything, you can go through with the course. Some courses might last a year but crash courses will last much lesser.

GET A LICENSE

The next thing is for you to get a license. You will need one to start your own business and without one, you might not be able to practice reflexology. Remember that you have to put it out on display so that people know you are qualified to perform the different reflexology techniques. Don't confuse the license with a degree certificate. You will need the former to open up a center and opening one without it might land you in trouble.

DEVIZE A PLAN

Once you get a license, you should work on a plan to open the center. The plan will help you take the next course of action with ease and you need not think too much for it. You have to write down how and when you will open the center, pick a place, decide on the financing etc. Planning all of it will help you have a smooth journey.

FIND A PLACE

Next, you must decide on an appropriate place for your business. As you know, you will need enough space to have a person lie down while you massage their feet or hands. You can either choose to convert your garage or a spare room in your house or rent a place for it. For the former option, you will have to take due permission for a commercial venture and carry out the business only if you are granted the permission. Starting with the practice without permission might land you in trouble. Once you finalize the place, you must move to the aspect of finance.

FINANCE

As you know, no business can function without proper finance. Therefore, you have to come up with enough financial resources to set up your center and also have some spare in case of an emergency. You can consider using your savings or apply for a loan from bank. You can also borrow from relatives or peers with a promise of returning it back with certain interested attached to it.

SET UP

The next step is for you to set up your business. You have to start by setting up the area where you wish to practice. You have to create a spa like environment replete with comfortable chairs, aromatherapy oils and candles, footbaths etc. You can also place some pamphlets that explain to people what reflexology is all about and what they can expect from your center. Once you set up your center, you must invite friends and family over to avail their feedback. You can make any requisite changes if they ask you to.

PRICING

You must then decide on the pricing. How you price the services will be based on the quality of the service. It will also be determined by how the others have priced their services. You can visit the other centers and collect their price pamphlets to see how they have priced the services that they provide at their centers. You must try and price it competitively but can provide an initial discount.

PRACTICE RUN

Next, you have to practice on as many people as possible before opening the center. Be it your family members or friends, you should try out the different techniques in order to see their response. It is obvious that they will give you a biased opinion but you must ask them to give you a genuine one on which you can plan your services.

OPEN CENTER

The next step is for you to open up your center. You have to advertise about it and inform as many people about it as possible. You can make use of social media to tell people about it or can also have pamphlets printed and posted. You should get your friends and family members to advertise as well and get word of your business put there. Your initial efforts will pay off in a big way.

EXPAND

You can decide to expand your business once you set it up. You can choose to increase the space and also start employing more people to join in. you can employ both reflexologists and also people to take care of your finances and attend to customers.

You can place televisions in the work areas which will show people how reflexology helps them in stimulating their body. The expansion plan and scale should be based on the resources that you have at your disposal.

These form the different steps that you have to take to start your own reflexology business. You will find it easy to open the business if you follow these steps in order. However, you can also use this as a blue print to start your own service.

CHAPTER 9

PRECAUTIONS TO BEAR IN MIND

DON'T APPLY TOO MUCH PRESSURE

It is important to ask about the pressure from time to time to ensure that it is appropriate. Too much pressure can cause unnecessary pain and you must keep adjusting the pressure from time to time.

DON'T STOP TREATMENT

If the patient is experiencing pain, then you must not abruptly stop the treatment. You can gently massage and complete the treatment fully before stopping it. If the patient is still in excess pain, then you can consider taking them to a physician. If you think it is just a sprain, then try applying a cold pack on the area.

MEALS

It is important to not provide treatment for at least an hour after having food and also an hour before food. Ask the patient when they had their last meal and give them the treatment based on their response.

WATER

It is extremely important to drink water after every treatment. Ask your patients to drink at least half a liter so that their bodies can remain well hydrated.

BONES/ VEINS

It is important for you to stay away from the bones and veins in the body as these are sensitive regions and you must not over stimulate them. Ask the patient if they are feeling any pressure on their bones and stop applying pressure immediately.

These form the different precautions that you must observe when it comes to providing reflexology. Remember safety comes first and you must be as careful as possible.

CHAPTER 10

WHO CAN IT HELP?

REFLEXOLOGY FOR CHILDREN AND ALSO INFANTS

Child Reflex is a mild type of reflexology produced particularly for children, babies as well as young children from one month to 3 years as it goes on and on.

Child Reflex is an amazing idea of Reflexology, which could boost the organic caring bond in between moms and dad and also kid, offering moms and dads the possibility to find out unique, mild, methods from a Reflexologist certified in Baby Reflex.

This calming type of finger-tip, as well as thumb stress, has been particularly developed for moms and dads to provide to their infants on their feet and also to their kids on their hands. Moms and dads could change the therapy to match their very own kid's demands.

Child Reflex was established by Jenny Lee, a Chartered Physiotherapist as well as certified Reflexologist, adhering to 15 years' considerable study into the results of routine Reflexology on Childhood Asthma. The primary results discovered in leisure, boosted rest and also child/parent bonding motivated Jenny to develop baby reflex in 2005.

Currently in 2014, Mums as well as Dads in Australia, South Africa, Abu Dhabi, Eire, Northern Ireland, Scotland, Wales, Japan, Turkey as well as Europe, offer the fuss-free, 5 min therapy of Baby Reflex, which intends to assist rest as well as boost wellness.

REFLEXOLOGY HOMEWORK TO HELP YOURSELF AT HOME

Not many people realize the subtle benefits of a good Reflexologist session. It's amazing the diverse improvements it can make to your well-being. Along with helping you heal and relieving pain, it can relieve the effects of stress, give a boost to your immune system, improve circulation, clear some of your body's toxins, relieve stress, and even assist in post-operative recovery by increasing blood to the immediate area. And the best thing about Reflexology is that it is so un-invasive. Without actually coming in contact with the area, that troubled are can be helped. But is there anything one can do after they have returned from a session with a Reflexologist to retain all those good benefits? There is a little homework you can do on your own.

TECHNIQUE

A registered Reflexologist practitioner will use their thumbs to exert mild pressure on the surface of the foot in a specific pattern during an actual Reflexology session. However, a focused massage with one of your hands on the opposite hand can be used to do a little follow-up and maintenance work from home. Often lumps, and under-the-skin deposits will be noticed to indicate where the problem lies. Also, sharper pain upon pressure will let you know if you are contacting the correct location on the area.

NECK AREA

The big toes on the feet and the thumbs on the hands relate to the neck area. If you face the thumb toward you, you will be able to discern the left side from the right. If your neck pain is on the right, you should massage up the length of the right side of the thumb. You will notice where there is a sore spot and you should concentrate on massaging that particular spot for a little while. Don't be afraid to apply pressure in and around the entire thumb, especially the outline of the thumb until you locate the painful or lumpy area. Massage for awhile until the pain decreases in the thumb area, even slightly.

SHOULDER AREA

The shoulder area is located on the lateral or outside, outline of the hand, just below the baby finger and also in a direct line from between the baby and the ring finger. A painful shoulder reflex usually shows up pretty quickly. Massage these painful areas and also the area down the top side of the baby finger.

KNEE AND SACROILIAC AREAS

These reflexology areas lie just below the outside shoulder area about mid-way down the outside or lateral part of the hand. Again a deep massage with the fingers of the other hand may reveal a painful spot that can be worked a little to aid the pain in the actual knee of sacroiliac areas.

LUMBAR VERTEBRAE

Turning the hand palm up will help you locate the lumbar/vertebrae reflex area of the back. It runs almost the entire length of the outside of the hand, where the thumb is located, when the hand is turned palm up. It starts just below the wrist and then runs up almost the entire thumb. If the palm was facing down this would be called the medial side of the hand. Massage up this entire length and you will be benefiting the lumbar area. Pay special attention to any painful areas.

SCIATIC AREA

The sciatic area is located on the wrist area about a half inch down from the bottom of the palm when it is turned- palm-side up. It runs a horizontal line right across the wrist and can be worked with the other hand. Massage right across the line. You may find some tender areas and it is recommended that you work these until the pain subsides slightly.

LUNG AREA

The lung area is situated on the palm-side of the hand, under the fingers and can actually continue on most of the palm's surface.

The most accessible area is under the fingers, concentrating on the first and second fingers. If you are suffering from any form of lung ailment or cold, it would be wise to work these areas in a general application. Chest colds, bronchitis, as well as other lung ailments will benefit from working this area.

HAND MASSAGE

It's a great idea to massage your entire hand in a deliberate and focused fashion searching for any sore or 'achy' areas. If you locate any spots that are sore and are not related to known hand pain, this could indicate a compromised area that relates to your body. If it is not actual hand pain, it is wise to massage this area until the pain dissipates.

BENEFITS OF HAND REFLEXOLOGY

- The hands are so much more accessible than the feet

- Hand reflexology can be quicker than foot reflexology

- It is so much more convenient

- It can be practiced in any locale

- The hands are closer to the spine so treatments can also help the central nervous system

There are very few body therapies that you can actually and effectively do on yourself. Although not as ideal as having a professional Reflexology session, helping yourself with your own hand Reflexology will still give you excellent results. It can aid in relieving common ailments such as frozen shoulder, mild back pain, neck pain from awkward sleeping and so much more. Your self-treatments can incorporate two or three reflex points so that you can work on them throughout the day- whenever you can to stimulate your body's own healing mechanisms.

With all the benefits and almost instant gratification one can feel from Reflexology and practicing on their own hands, it is a wise suggestion to give it a try. The relaxation benefit alone is worth having a professional session by a registered Reflexologist. It also may be worthwhile to familiarize oneself with all the associated reflexes of the hand to be able to help yourself as much as you can with any pain and/or problems that may arise.

REFLEXOLOGY FOR FERTILITY

Reflexology therapies have often been proclaimed as an ideal treatment for trying to conceive. Although many have dismissed reflexology as a worthless and useless means of treatment, there is evidence to suggest otherwise.

WHAT IS REFLEXOLOGY?

Reflexology is a complimentary treatment which utilizes massage of the feet in order to stabilize and balance the body. There is evidence that the origins of reflexology lay in ancient China, Greece and Egypt within a few years of each other but it is has only been structured into a more organized treatment within the last several decades.

The treatment uses a more natural means to heal the body, founded upon the notion that certain points, or meridians, within the feet are connected to internal organs within the rest of the body. It is believed that when these points are touched and stimulated, then certain areas of the body will feel beneficial effects.

WILL IT HELP ME GET PREGNANT?

Reflexology practitioners believe that by using certain massage techniques on the feet they are able to remove the body of particular toxins within the body, allowing enhanced circulation to take place and allowing the endocrine system, which produces the hormones, to come back into balance and overall aid fertility.

In addition to this, reflexology is believed to help in reducing the amount of stress a couple can experience when trying to achieve conception – this includes lack of sleep, appetite, tension and stress. Reflexology can help reduce these annoying side effects of trying to create a baby.

There have been certain studies which have studied how reflexology has improved the impact of trying to conceive a baby; however, it should be stressed that there is not a lot of official medical research done on the subject. There are some studies which have suggested that some alternative therapies can reduce fertility, whereas there are others which suggest that reflexology and other natural therapies can actually aid a woman in getting pregnant.

As a result, although there is the suggestion that reflexology can help in getting you pregnant, it is still unknown whether it can help you conceive. It is more likely that it aids a couple in getting pregnant by helping the women reduce the amount of stress she is experiencing, helping to improve on the amount of sleep she is getting, improving the appetite etc., which makes her body more receptive to creating the right environment of holding onto a baby. However, it should be stressed that there is no 100% guarantee that reflexology will work, but if you are open to these kinds of alternative therapies then it is well worth trying it.

WHAT DOES A TREATMENT INVOLVE?

When you begin your treatment, your reflexology practitioner will initially discuss your current and general health, whether you are undergoing any treatments, taking any medication or what other issues you may have. Then they will look and touch your feet.

Your reflexology practitioner will determine what areas are experiencing the most tension and will focus on these areas in order to unblock energy in the related area of your body. However, your reflexology practitioner will typically work on the entire foot in order to bring your body back into balance.

Reflexology treatments will typically take an hour and your practitioner will discuss with you a course of treatment in order for you to get the best results for your needs.

REFLEXOLOGY DURING PREGNANCY AND LABOR: LABOR TRIGGER POINTS EXPLAINED

Reflexology books and programs are typically rather unclear on the topic of pregnancy, thinking that only 'skilled Reflexologists must deal with pregnant women; they emphasis the concern of potential miscarriages and the verity that therapy may well have unforeseen consequences. It is correct that it's not dangerous to start treatment once the 12th week has finished and providing the woman hasn't experienced miscarriages or bleeding as it is this is that there are particular positions on the bottom of the foot that once pushed may possibly activate childbirth. It is as a result dangerous to motivate such areas in the beginning of your pregnancy, for they can cause miscarriage.

In contrast, reflexology can be the perfect treatment for the duration of pregnancy – this isn't just because it is absolutely soothing and has a harmonizing result on both the body and passions; furthermore, as a useful aspect, as the pregnant mother will not be required to lay down flat on her back as if she would have to do if she was being massaged (sitting upwards can be done if wanted), and reflexology can be effortlessly implemented, nearly all over. The rationalization why retrieving energy and motivating precise zones is successful as a general balancer is because the bottom of the feet is an 'active plan' of the entire body. For example, in acupuncture terms, all of the meridians throughout the body 'finishes' on the bottom of the foot, so encouraging an area on the bottom of the foot will habitually - actively speaking – opening numerous further energy areas, and touching quite a lot of organs. Reflexology is likewise perfect for 'mingling' with additional therapies, including Reiki, all things which are safe to use in pregnancy.

Reflexology practitioners claim that it is not impossible to observe the head of the infant on the base of feet of the pregnant mother: that is to say matching to the zone of the bladder (which is actually some of the parts that requires massaging in order to bring about labor). Reflexology is extraordinary as a supplement and as an implement to actively sort out the imbalance between the mind and the body, as an understated and entirely rounded means; on the other hand allopathic treatment is the leading treatment regarding diagnostics. As a result, it is extremely central to ensure with the family doctor and anyone else dealing with you during the pregnancy, to be in no doubt that there aren't any primary complications which could exacerbate from the practice of reflexology.

There are certainly areas which should be left alone before getting to full term (which means not before the 37th week of your pregnancy), as these areas could induce labor. Reflexology 'unlocks conduits': they have a dynamic influence on your body due to the fact that they fortify the body's capacity to deal with contractions, but in addition to this, they have a balancing influence as the pregnant woman is mindful of the fact that her body is prepared to deal with this significant event.

The beginning of labor (known as parturition in medical terminology) is caused through an intricate collaboration hormones which includes estrogen. This causes the neck of the womb to slowly but surely widen and as a final point 'push out the baby. This miracle is quite a natural one, something the body does on its own without any help from others at times, nevertheless is the principal impediments to a quick birth (providing there aren't any key bodily issues) is the mother's own subliminal fear, which single-handedly can impede the consistent distribution of the correct hormones, which means the necessary energy needed for labor and the birth is removed.

It is not an accident that hypnotherapy birth courses recently experienced a high deal of attention and popularity amongst mothers from all around the world. Pregnant mothers are now coming to the realization that in today's culture we have turned out to be detached from what our bodies are trying to tell us and it is for that reason the trouble with appealing with things as ordinary as childbirth, breast-feeding and the overall 'chaos' that it entails.

However, the body is well aware of what is required of it and modern medicine is always there to support us if it becomes necessary. However, the healing art of reflexology can benefit us by allowing the pregnant mother to communicate within herself: releasing energy through channels, to make her body get ready for the complicated development of birth.

Important reflexology areas are those which are related to the release of hormones, with the pituitary and thyroid glands being the principal ones. It is these areas which require being pushed in quite a firm manner. Labor is controlled through the release of the hormone oxytocin being created. The pituitary is situated upon the biggest toe. Hormones essential for the creation of breast milk consist of insulin and several other hormones. As a result, you will need to encourage the thyroid and parathyroid area, so that your body experiences an additional increase in getting ready for when baby finally emerges out of the body. This particular area is positioned in the middle of the biggest toe and the index toe. Some maps claim that this area is linked with your cerebellum, which the primary task is generally governing the motor skills structure, although it should be stressed that there are suggestions though that this section has other occupations, which includes learning.

The zone conforming to the bladder requires a firm stimulating motion in order to encourage the beginning of labor. The central chest zone is in what is referred to as the 'power' region and stimulating this region has a general harmonizing and soothing result. Reflexology practitioners say that in addition to this, that your emotional heart is located here, essential for pregnant women who are scared to go into labor.

Important parts are likewise those parallel to the ovary and the womb, mainly a location in the vicinity which rests in the hollow close to the malleolus. This region is tremendously sensitive near the end of pregnancy and requires firmly pressing again and again, but the results are worth it. Many women will experience false labor but this emphasizes the fact that it should not be done during the early part of your pregnancy. Last of all, acupressure recommends that you push strongly on the smallest toe and on its side as it's a connection to the bladder channel.

Bodies will jump into action when the body tells it is time, so using pressure on the points gives the body encouragement but it should be stated that they are amazingly successful in helping the body release the necessary hormones required for childbirth. Reflexology on the hands can likewise be useful, effectual just as reflexology on the feet is. Altogether the areas which have been explained before can be located in equivalent positions - the pituitary, uterus, bladder etc. Hand reflexology is far more useful as it involves extremely minor planning and could be practiced at practically no matter what the time or location. Furthermore, you should definitely concentrate on the shoulders and the surrounding area as there is an area in the middle of the necks and the shoulders - should you apply pressure in an extremely firm manner – such as with the elbow - has the ability to bring on labor! You can still enjoy massages in this region but it should be done in a gentle manner.

From looking at the information above, we can see that reflexology can be great during your pregnancy. It can have an influence on the entire body through means of an energetic manner instead of just through a physical means. By applying the appropriate amount of pressure on certain areas of the body, you can unblock certain channels which can build up through various different emotional means that can, in turn, have an influence within yourself.

REFLEXOLOGY

Reflexology is known to most of the world as an "alternative medicine." Even though it is typically used in combination with traditional medical treatment, some people choose to use it instead of medical treatment, which is not recommended.

Reflexology involves applying pressure to various places in the feet, hands and face to achieve a desired result. The pressure points in reflexology are determined by a system of zones and reflex areas that are reported to be directly connected to other locations on the human body. These points are reported to cause a physical or chemical change in the body. There is no medical evidence that reflexology itself can treat any medical condition. However, there is evidence that reflexology, when combined with other medical sciences, can be extremely beneficial to the treatment of patients from various backgrounds.

HOW CAN I FIND A REFLEXOLOGIST?

Reflexology is not officially regulated at this time so it is essential that you choose your reflexology practitioner carefully and wisely. It is important that whoever you chose to treat you is someone that you are comfortable with because if you are not then it could reduce the amount of benefits you will gain throughout your treatment.

When choosing a reflexology practitioner it is best to go with someone that has been recommended to you by someone whom you trust. However, there are a number of organizations that can help you find a reflexology practitioner in your locality. These include the Association of Reflexologists, the British Complementary Therapy Association and the British Reflexology Association.

As with any treatment, it is important that you discuss reflexology with your doctor before you start having treatment.

WHAT HAPPENS IN A REFLEXOLOGY SESSION?

The therapist always begins with them conducting a brief health history on the client in question. They are trying to determine which reflexology therapy might be the best choice for you and your needs.

It is okay to ask questions while the intake is being conducted. A therapist wants you to feel comfortable with communication and the session in itself. A red flag will appear if you as the client feel the therapist isn't being completely honest with you. This shouldn't be taken lightly and the session should be ended immediately.

HOW DOES A TYPICAL SESSION START?

Your specific health issues will determine which area the therapist decides to work on first. The situation at hand will also determine which area is best to work on. For example, if you are in the hospital hooked up to machines, the feet will better accessible to the reflexologist. You will either be standing or lying down. No matter what area is being performed on, the client will always be clothes unless shoes and socks are being removed to work on the feet.

The treatment will be determined whether or not there are injuries or open wounds. A session usually lasts no more than an hour long. You do not have to talk during a session but resting is an option to. Feedback is always important to give to your practitioner, and you can always tell them to stop at any given time. It is your right to do so.

WHAT IS THE FOCUS OF THE SESSION?

Whether you have any health conditions or not, reflexology therapy revolves around the entire pattern starting at the toes and working down the entire foot. A practitioner will take extra care with specific conditions. They will be sure to work all the areas of the foot with a pressure that is gentle. The nerve pathways and congestion help release and promotes relaxation to the entire body.

If you suffer from migraines, then those specific points in

relation to the migraine will be worked to release those tension and sensations to create relaxation. The entire pattern of a foot can address all of the body.

WHAT IS REFLEXOLOGY TREATMENT?

Different techniques will include all of the points on each foot, maybe even the hands or ears. Fingers and toes are usually the starting point and is worked down to the base of limb. The sides and tops are worked in movements alongside the entire body component.

When all the points are being worked in unison, the internal organs and glands and etc are being worked as well. This includes the nerves and bone groups too. Pressure is applied when only the reflexologist finds any type of congestion or tightness in the session. This pressure will allow the body to come back into a balance of unison. Harmony is brought to the body when an area is full of pain. The release of pain is not their motto. However, the goal is to bring the body into harmony and a balance.

A therapist isn't there to fix it but to stimulate the body such as the nervous system to do all the work. They will often return to the spot to confirm the once felt pain has been released.

WHAT WILL A CLIENT EXPERIENCE DURING A SESSION?

No one has the same experience during a reflexology session. The key to a successful therapy session is to gain a sense of relaxation and to bring awareness to the internal area of the body while it is being worked. Clients often feel a tingling or lightness in their bodies. It is warm and comforting as they feel the energy flowing their body at normal pace. They can often feel it through each organ, gland or even muscle. There are other reactions such as perspiration in the area, sensation of cold or feeling chilled and/or laughing. Each reaction is different for each client.

Reflexologists do not diagnose clients. They do however, repeat sessions. A therapist cannot and will not tell you about any condition or tension while working on you during a session. They may suggest abnormalities though.

WHAT HAPPENS AT THE END OF THE SESSION?

Stroking is often a type of sensation of calm they revoke on their clients. It leaves them feeling cared and nurtured. The practitioner tells you to pay attention to your body and how it reacts after a session. Sometimes a person is recommended to drink water or to even rest. The reaction your body gives you will tell you how to treat yourself after a session. A practitioner should be called only if the reactions to a session are concerning you.

It has been known that clients have increased energy, relief from pain as well enhanced sleep. Each reaction is different for each person. These are not the only benefits people tend to experience afterwards.

HOW MANY SESSIONS ARE NEEDED?

Reflexology therapist cannot tell you many sessions are required to make you feeling better. The health of the client and for the reasons you wanted to do reflexology in the first place. The sessions may need to be more frequent if you are dealing with a specific condition or illness. Sometimes clients will do one session a week for six to eight weeks. Than after they can do a follow up appointment every four weeks. It all depends on how your body is and reacts to the treatments.

In conclusion, the client is the only one who can determine if reflexology therapy is best for them. A therapist and the client will work together to create a plan that best fits the needs of the person. Reflexology has helped a lot of people to release stress and tension from their bodies. It has allowed these clients to have a better life expectancy and to live healthier.

CHAPTER 11

TRAINING AND EDUCATION

Reflexology is tutored through a collection of workshops, courses, and also training movies. Qualification is gained after a 6-month plan that consists of 200 hours of training. The credentials of training can be subdivided into various aspects which include: 28 hours of initial workshop training; 14 hours of sophisticated workshop training; 58 hours of self-directed research study; and also 100 hours of practical encounter, consisting of providing reflexology to a minimum of 15 individuals.

Particular facets of the training consist of direction in the analysis of the stress factors on the feet as well as hands via a research of human composition. Pupils additionally discover how to offer reflexology sessions to individuals together with certain strategies for dealing with the hands.

CERTIFICATION AND ADVANCED CERTIFICATION

The independently American Reflexology Certification Board (ARCB) licenses the expertise of reflexology experts on a specific basis. Requirements for specific accreditation consist of the end of academic needs as well as passing a conventional certifying examination.

Minimum certification to take the credentials exam involves being present at an innovative workshop within two years before taking the assessment. Furthermore, the candidate needs to have gone to initial workshops for two complete days along with the needed day of innovative workshop training, as well as the candidate is required to have a minimum of 6 months of useful experience in carrying out the treatment. Applicants are checked out through both created examinations as well as useful presentation.

Advanced training concentrates on understanding the capability to execute hand reflexology. Some reflexology training courses might be used in various other course fields, depending on the particular program of research as well as the credentials of the individual training organizations included.

MEDICAL USES

There were numerous reviews and journal articles released between the years of 2009 and 2011 that provide more than enough evidence supporting reflexology as a secondary form of treatment for various medical conditions, especially chronic, long-term and terminal illnesses. In 2009, a systematic review of multiple controlled trials that are based on reflexology, demonstrate that it is in fact effective in assisting with various medical procedures, including cancer therapy.

As a result of these studies, many governments are trying to push health insurance companies to cover treatments when they are being used for treatment of certain illnesses and injuries.

REGULATION

There are very few places where reflexology is regulated by any specific board or facility. For example, in the UK, reflexologists are registered on a voluntary basis. However, in order to be registered, the facility or person must meet certain Standards of Proficiency that have been outlined by specific boards, such as the CNHC. Currently, there are only 14 reflexologists registered with the CNHC, but there were not very many applications either.

In Canada, reflexology is not regulated by any specific board or group. They have also made mention that reflexology bills do not qualify as insurance claims and they cannot be used on income taxes as medical bills. The Reflex Association of Canada does provide a listing of all reflexologists who choose to register themselves as a business.

In the United States, there are several certification boards that a reflexologist may join if they choose. These boards are non-profit organizations that are attempting to increase the standards that have been set for reflexologists and attempting to demand more education and licensing regulations for patient safety.

The advantage to becoming a member of one of these certification boards is that you have the ability to prove that you are skilled in reflexology and that you are not just a fly-by-night person who decided it looked fun.

Reflexology and Medical Treatment

Reflexology is an elective procedure that uses the hands, feet, face and ears to help increase the overall well-being of the human body. In total, there are 45 techniques that are used on various reflex points.

When combined with medical treatment, reflexology encourages the body to heal; it does not actually MAKE it heal.

THE PURPOSE OF REFLEXOLOGY

· It helps to reduce the effects that stress and tension have on the body.

· It helps improve nerve conduction, circulation and lymphatic circulation

· It helps to normalize the balance of the body systems, which is called homeostasis.

HOW DOES REFLEXOLOGY WORK?

· Each hand and foot contains approximately 7,200 nerves, which creates at least 200,000 nerve endings in each hand and foot.

- Pressure is applied to a group of nerve endings, which is what is referred to as a reflex point.

- The nerve cluster is alerted that pressure has been applied and a signal is sent to the brain.

- At times, the brain responds to this signal with pain.

- The body then mobilizes due to the response and begins the healing process on its own.

WHAT REFLEXOLOGY CAN AND CANNOT DO

- Reflexology is considered a non-invasive therapy, but is considered a persuasive therapy. There are not very many contraindications to reflexology, meaning it cannot cause health problems.

- Reflexology CAN reduce the amount of stress and tension that is felt in the body. Reduced stress and tension lead to increased circulation, lymphatic drainage, and help break down and eliminate the toxins found in the body. This strengthens the immune system and reduces the risk of a secondary infection in those who are at risk.

- Reflexology is sometimes used by doctors to indicate where higher areas of tension and stress are in the body. By relieving this stress and tension through physiotherapy, the doctor may be able to reduce the amount of pain medication their patient is on and promote the natural healing process.

- Reflexology has been proven to help treat chronic and acute injuries and illnesses.

- Reflexologists CANNOT diagnose injuries, illnesses or conditions because they are not medical doctors.

- Reflexology SHOULD NOT be substituted for medical treatment. It is a complementary treatment that is meant to accompany the supervision of a licensed medical professional.

- Reflexology CAN NOT decrease, increase, over-stimulate or alter any way that the body functions. This means that it cannot be dangerous.

THE PRINCIPLES OF REFLEXOLOGY

Reflexology is a fascinating ancient science that is built on the principle that reflexes and an extremely effective form of therapeutic foot massage that relates to the internal organs and other structures of the body. Reflexology is regarded as both science and art; as a science because it is based on neurological and physiological studies and as an art as much of it depends on the skills of the therapist and their own knowledge.

The feet are just one part of the body but they are ultimately connected to the rest of the body. All the body parts, including the glands and organs, are represented by reflexes in a particular sequence on the feet. Their positions and relationships to each other follow a rational, anatomical order which closely resembles that of the body itself.

The technique that is used for reflexology is the "thumb or finger", which stimulates the nerve endings, allowing any energy blockages to be released, thereby causing physiological changes to take place in the body. Hence, its science states that where there is sensitivity in a reflex position, there is an indication of stress or weakness in the corresponding organ or body part.

Reflexology aims to trigger the return of homeostasis in the body; a state of equilibrium or balance. This step is best achieved by reducing tension and inducing relaxation. Relaxation is the first approach to normalization and healing is possible when the body is relaxed. When the blood vessels are not constricted, circulation is considerably enhanced and each cell in the body can be properly supplied with nutrients and oxygen. The body's organs can work normally.

An excellent treatment can take up to 45 minutes to be completed. All reflexes are stimulated by a stimulating a specific sequence by the therapist, considering any sensitivity or pain. Congested molecules that are formed at the nerve endings are all broken down by the treatment (72,000 each foot) and the healing process begins.

THE ANCIENT CHINESE MERIDIANS

The Meridians system was discovered by the Chinese around 3,000 years ago and since then the idea has gone from strength to strength to become developed and researched science today.

The Meridians are known for electrical pathways or networks of energy covering the body that are identical to the zones that are traditionally referred to as reflexology. There are twelve main Meridians or invincible channels, with each passing through one side of the body and having a similar image on the other side.

A simple knowledge of the Meridians can help a therapist understand the diseased pathways and help them in locating the problem areas. 'Chi' is the energy running through the Meridians. This energy is gotten from the food we eat and the air we breathe, both of which are considered to be the 'fruit of life', the important energy within the body that nourishes body and mind. To enhance a healthy living and chi, individuals should engage in a healthy diet, exercise, healthy breathing exercises, good posture and limited stress. Hence, a poor diet, poor breathing, lack of exercise, poor posture and excess stress will drain the chi, thereby causing an internal imbalance that may result in disease.

Evidence will be felt in the form of congestions along the pathways when the Meridians are running on a low current. These congestions are diagnostic conditions that some people suffer from, such as sinus problems, breast lumps, constipation, headaches and knee pains.

A closer view of the Meridians shows that there are six main

Meridians found in the feet, specifically the toes; the Meridians will touch the main organs – stomach, liver, spleen/pancreas, gallbladder, bladder and kidneys. Treatment on reflexology will stimulate and clear congestions along all these Meridians, thereby allowing the free flow of energy and return of the body to a state of balance.

There are certain conditions and evidence that should be looked at such as bunions, plantar warts, corns, calluses and nail conditions and congestions along the Meridians in question. These problems should be looked upon by the therapist in other to teach their patients about the underlying causes and encourage them to take full responsibility of their lifestyle changes.

For example, a disorder in the stomach Meridian may cause upper toothache as the Meridian passes through the upper gums. Lower toothache may be as a result of a disorder of the large intestine Meridian. The Meridians can be used to effectively provide a better knowledge of the conditions affecting the body.

QUANTUM PHYSICS OF THE HUMAN BODY

Quantum physics identifies the interplay of many energetic pressures that combine to form a whole. The human body is basically a changing process and health is the balance of energy in reaction to the body's internal and external environments. The above theory is correct when analyzing the logical progression of the structural levels of molecules, cells and organs. However, beyond the structural level of molecules, mechanical becomes less and now enters the world governed by probability, unpredictable action and energy.

For centuries, we have solicited professional advice to understand the science behind the colors in the feet that come after a Vacuflex Concepts boot treatment. Scientists have given the answer consistently that the colors display a thermal energy.

The sun is the major source of thermal energy that is available to mankind and it supplies the earth with the all-important light and heat. At a primary level, thermal energy comes from the variation of atoms and molecules in matter. It is a form of kinetic energy developed from the random variations of those molecules when the thermal energy of a system can be increased or decreased.

The increased variation of the molecules in the reflex areas on the feet could be a result of the exerted pressure to the reflex areas by thumb and finger techniques during the treatment, or could be the negative vacuum pressure by the Vacuflex concept body treatment.

Some years ago, photos of a pair of feet were taken with an infrared camera before and after reflexology treatment was performed. Comprehensive evidence of thermal energy in the whole body is shown by comparing the before and after photos.

RESEARCH PROBLEMS

As with any type of therapy, there has been some research into what possible problems could arise from undergoing reflexology, or any other alternative therapy for that matter. Let us now take a look at some of the concerns healthcare professionals may have in regards to reflexology.

Potential Problem Number One

It is simply impossible to substantiate the claim that reflexology has in regards to prevention or curing of diseases or health problems. In order to prove this, there would have to be controlled clinical trials which would consist of several years of systematic testing using hundreds of patients and cost a fortune. This is in addition to any moral issues that could arise from testing patients with actual pain or health issues. It would mean that sick people, those that experience pain, would not be allowed to take normal medical care and it is important that we do not deprive patients of the right medical attention. Despite this, however, reflexology practitioners are believed to be able to determine health issues that medical doctors already know about.

Potential Problem Number Two

It is well known amongst the healthcare industry that patients will give doctors (and other healthcare providers) the information that they have. People will certainly talk about their bodily issues with anyone who gives them a listening ear. However, it is believed that reflexology practitioners could determine any health issues simply by listening to patients ramble on about themselves and as a result, this means that should reflexology actually be tested in a clinical way, the patients and practitioners would not be allowed to communicate with each other. Certain words, such as "ow", "that does hurt", "a little", "a lot", "yes", "No" etc. would be allowed in a clinical trial as although this may seem a little cold, it would mean that the reflexology practitioner would not be able to discern existing medical conditions from the patient through talking with one another.

Potential Problem Number Three

There is another way that patients communicate with doctors and healthcare workers known as subliminal cuing. This means that they communicate without recognizing what they are actually doing. This is also referred to as body language or muscle reading. If reflexology was to be conducted in a controlled clinical trial in order to determine the benefits of the alternative therapy then it would mean that the patient and the reflexology practitioner would have to separated through some sort of curtain or veil so that the reflexology practitioner should not be able to see what the patient is telling them subconsciously or through the way their body talks.

WHAT ARE THE DANGERS OF REFLEXOLOGY?

Many people are hesitant in beginning courses of treatment such as reflexology as they do not know if there are any dangers to it. I am happy to confirm that reflexology does not have any direct way to cause a patient harm but it should be stressed that you should not use reflexology in order to prevent or cure any existing or potential health issues. If you have any concerns it is vital that you seek out qualified medical assistance through your general practitioner.

The biggest danger when it comes to reflexology is the belief that it can diagnose any and every health issue you could face. It cannot do this. Do not use reflexology as your only means of medical therapy. It is essential that you realize that reflexology practitioners are not qualified medical doctors and there have been cases in the past, such as Rosalie Tarpening, that have had conflicts with the law regarding her capabilities. Tarpening had a certificate from a university which had closed down and she went on to develop her services beyond midwifery into more alternative healthcare practices. This led to her being convicted of 2nd degree murder of an infant who was stillborn in 1989. The pregnant mother pleaded with Tarpening to allow her to go to hospital but she refused, saying that childbirth was easy and natural. Because of her lack of knowledge and her incapability to understand the seriousness of the circumstances, it led to the death of an innocent and healthy baby and the mother having to experience regret and anger at herself for the rest of her life.

THE RAA OFFERS RELEASED CRITERIA OF TECHNIQUE FOR REFLEXOLOGISTS.

There are some various concepts on just how reflexology functions:

Chi power: This notion is based upon the suggestion that reflexology stabilizes the circulation of energy (chi) in the body, which causes recovery.

Counter irritation: The body reacts to health problem or injury with an immune feedback. Some reflexologists think that the body regularly aims to bring back stability. Furthermore, reflexology successfully develops an "injury," creating the body to look for equilibrium.

Crystalline deposits: It accumulates in the feet gradually. Reflexologists think that these deposits obstruct nerve closings as well as reduce the circulation of power throughout the body. Reflexologist's damage down these deposits, which they think makes it possible for the body to recover itself by introducing obstructed power.

Lymph water drainage: The body's lymphatic tract gets rid of excess liquid and also toxic substances from the body. Some reflexologists assert that reflexology boosts the lymphatic tract, enhancing its general feature and also consequently removing even more toxic substances.

Electrical response: Some reflexologists think that the body is comprised of various sorts of electric impulses. It could create an inequality somewhere else in the body if one impulse is subduing the others. Reflexology, in their perspective, assists rebalances the body's electric impulses as well as brings about recovery.

Psychological response: Some reflexologists think that the mind plays a huge part in encouraging the body that it has recovered. They believe that reflexology produces an effective inactive medicine impact.

Proprioception: Reflexologists that credit this concept say that reflexology cues the peripheral nervous system to send out the body incorrect messages that the body has been rebalanced. Subsequently, the human brain sends out signals to loosen up the muscular tissues, which brings about recovery

CONCLUSION

I thank you once again for choosing this book and hope you had a good time reading it.

The main aim of this book was to educate you on the meaning, method and benefits of reflexology.

As you can see, it is quite simple for you to take up the practice and exploit it. You will feel like a new person, once you start availing the massages.

You don't have to be a qualified reflexologist to perform some of the massages. However, you might have to exercise a little precaution and try to remain within limits to prevent any injuries.

If you experience pain or any other unpleasant sensation, then you must immediately make your way to a doctor and have him or her check it out.

As we saw in the last chapter, once you get your degree, you can consider opening up your own reflexology center.

I wish you luck with your reflexology endeavors and hope you experience great relief.

All the best!

Printed in Great Britain
by Amazon